The Moon in the Water

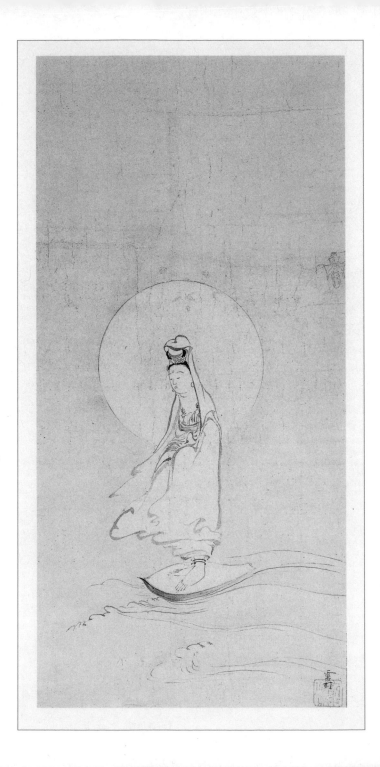

The Moon in the Water

REFLECTIONS ON AN AGING PARENT

Kathy J. Phillips

VANDERBILT UNIVERSITY PRESS   NASHVILLE

11 10 09 08   1 2 3 4 5

This book is printed on acid-free paper
made from 50% post-consumer recycled paper.
Manufactured in the United States of America

Frontispiece: "One-petal Kannon," or "The Bodhisattva
Kannon Crossing the Sea on a Lotus Petal," by Zen artist
Sesson Shūkei (1504–1589?), courtesy of the Alsdorf
collection.
Jacket design by Louise OFarrell
Text design by Dariel Mayer

Library of Congress Cataloging-in-Publication Data

Phillips, Kathy J., 1950-
The moon in the water : reflections on an aging parent /
Kathy J. Phillips. 1st ed.
p. cm.
ISBN 978-0-8265-1586-5 (cloth)
1. Aging parents—Care—Anecdotes. 2. Adult children
of aging parents—Anecdotes. 3. Caregivers—Anecdotes.
4. Parent and adult child—Anecdotes. 5. Avalokitesvara
(Buddhist deity)—Art—Miscellanea. I. Title.
HQ1063.6.P48 2008
306.874084'609969-dc22
2007026255

Contents

Preface

These vignettes record the interactions, wary and warm, of an elderly father and a middle-aged daughter living in the same house after many years of independence. Each vignette describes a painting of the Water-Moon Kuan Yin type in Buddhist art, then ventures into some trial facing the new housemates, then interweaves the painting and the life.

In Buddhism, Kuan Yin is a bodhisattva, or enlightened soul, who has incarnated many times and could graduate from the round of births and deaths but instead chooses to keep incarnating, to help others. In art, she has maybe a dozen different, typical poses: sitting on a bench with one knee drawn up, standing and pouring her water jar of spiritual sustenance. I only developed an interest in the particular pose called Water-Moon after my dad moved in; in these pictures, Kuan Yin does nothing but sit on a tiny island or jutting embankment and watch for the reflection of the moon in the water. Did I suddenly notice her because I was feeling a little confined as caregiver? Was my dad maybe feeling confined too: plunked on an island (O'ahu, Hawai'i), marooned in a doctor's office, belted into a wheelchair, locked in illness, backed into old age? Yet

Kuan Yin manages to be perfectly content on her precarious ledge. *How in the world does she do it?*

You don't really need any more information than that about Kuan Yin to read this memoir about caregiving; you could skip right away to the vignettes. For anybody who wants more background, the Chinese name Kuan Yin or Guanyin means "the one who perceives the sound of suffering," a rough translation of the Sanskrit name Avalokitesvara. Although Indian Buddhists depicted Avalokitesvara as male, his stories underwent a transformation as they passed into China. From the seventh to the ninth centuries, Chinese Buddhists may have combined the legends of this Indian bodhisattva of compassion with those of Tara, a Tantric female figure, or with the stories of the Taoist Queen Mother of the West.[1] Her differently pronounced names include Goon Yum in Cantonese, Kannon in Japanese, Quan Im in Thai, and Quan Am in Vietnamese. With the exceptions of the male Kwanseum in Korea and Chenrezig in Tibet, Asia today predominantly represents Kuan Yin as a woman.

I learned about Kuan Yin in 1977 after I moved to Hawai'i. A resident can easily spot this bodhisattva, not only at the Honolulu Academy of Arts but also at outdoor shrines, a mural on a building, a laminated picture dangling from a knapsack, and temples from multiple cultures.[2] Although I completed a Ph.D. in comparative literature, I have always been a closet religion major. A singer in the Hindu *Upanishads* comes up with a series of beautiful comparisons for the highest god—"like a flame of fire," "like a saffron-colored robe"—but after each phrase, the singer has to admit, "not this, not this." Nevertheless, the list goes on, because, the text insists, we *need* provisional words and images to help us begin to understand. I also discovered that Hinduism tolerantly accepts very different "yogas" or paths to union with the divine. (The English word *yoking* or union comes from the same root as *yoga*.) Some people do better by going to the mountaintop and meditating on a formless god, while others need a personal dialogue with a god in a clear, human-like form. This personalized path is called "bhakti" or devotional yoga. For me, the interesting point is that Hinduism recognizes the provisional, not absolute quality of the different routes to the divine. Even the gods of Hinduism are marked out as stepping-stones: the best our human minds can come up with for a time, to get a little closer to something greater than all human words and images.

I am attracted to bhakti or personalized devotion as it appears in various world religions—always with the understanding that the particular visualization is a tentative, imperfect, human construct. The thirteenth-century poet Jelaluddin Rumi, practicing Sufism (a mystical branch of Islam), calls his god "the Friend" and speaks right up to him in a personal, cheeky, and (at least in translations by Coleman Barks) very down-to-earth dialogue. In a mystical branch of Judaism, where god is not the more familiar, all-powerful Yahweh but a being who weeps when we don't accept happiness from him, the eighteenth-century Baal Shem Tov advises us to get busy and "dance" god into the world.[3] And though Buddhism, which grew out of Hinduism, abolished any gods, those Buddhist sects that developed bodhisattvas offered their worshipers a functional equivalent of a bhakti-type devotion. These bodhisattvas aren't exterior saviors sitting on some cloud somewhere but an inner ideal: "by the practice of meditation the lake of the heart becomes pure and calm . . . it is the reflection of a Bodhisattva which appears within it."[4]

The reason that Kuan Yin stood out for me as a possible visualization toward something spiritual in myself is simply that many artworks and legends picture her as a woman. By contrast, Islam and Judaism have preserved primarily male poets singing to male gods. Hinduism has a few more female devotee/poets—the twelfth-century Mahādēviyakka and the sixteenth-century Mirabai—but they usually pine for male gods, Shiva or Krishna. Within Christianity, Mary intercedes for her worshippers, but she is clearly a secondary figure. Kuan Yin is one of the few figures in world religions who does not gain her place of dignity as someone else's mother or daughter or consort.

Although it appeals to me that my primary teaching figure be a woman, I should emphasize that I do not believe that compassion is a particularly feminine trait, as some Westerners studying Kuan Yin in the 1950s assumed. Ancient Indian Buddhists held that a bodhisattva of

The Moon in the Water

compassion could *only* incarnate in a man. Americans in the 1950s (drawing on a nineteenth-century gendered division of labor) held the opposite idea: that a bodhisattva of compassion would *naturally* incarnate as a woman. The contradiction in these two views teaches us that *both* conceptions are social, not natural at all. The more modern way of assigning compassion to women or to a so-called "feminine side" of men may cause men to think it's not quite "right" for them to be kind. Such a misconception may lead boys to hide kindness or push them toward soldiering just to prove a spurious manliness. In caregiving, the odd gendered divisions into either "feminine" caring, on the one hand, or "masculine" force or rationality, on the other, have also stiflingly prevented men, until recently, from entering the nursing professions.

To anchor my experience with my dad, I start each vignette about him by describing an actual, specific painting of Water-Moon Kuan Yin, which I have seen in a book, journal article, or the occasional traveling exhibit at the Honolulu Academy of Arts. At the end of this volume, I acknowledge all these sources in a list, keyed to the vignettes. Some of the original pictures show a female Water-Moon Kuan Yin, some a male. Usually I regularize the descriptions to a female Kuan Yin, to indicate that a female teacher is important to me. But this gender bias isn't a hard and fast rule. Occasionally I keep to the original painting's male Kuan Yin. Moreover, people of both sexes in the vignettes—friends, known neighbors, mere elevator acquaintances, or strangers in the street who helped us out—also stand in for Kuan Yin, taking over the roles from the paintings. After all, the whole point is that anyone is potentially a bodhisattva.[5]

Finally, at the end of this volume, I offer a short summary of different meanings (as best I can see them) that have been assigned to Water-Moon imagery over the centuries. I put off that page until an afterword, so that you, reader, have a chance to make meanings for yourself from the art and the life.

NOTES

1   Diana Y. Paul, "Kuan-yin: Savior and Savioress in Chinese Pure Land Buddhism," in *The Book of the Goddess Past and Present*, ed. Carl Olson (New York: Crossroad, 1983), 174.

2   For more information on Kuan Yin, see the introduction to my earlier book of poems, placing Kuan Yin in the muck and muddle of every day, *This Isn't a Picture I'm Holding: Kuan Yin* (Honolulu: University of Hawai'i Press, 2004). To recognize Kuan Yin in artworks, the surest signs are a jar, a willow branch, and a raised portion over the forehead (in a topknot or headdress), which either pictures the Buddha or leaves a blank space.

3   Quoted in Annie Dillard, *For the Time Being* (New York: Vintage-Random, 1999), 137, 144.

4   Quoted in Edward Conze, ed. and trans., *Buddhist Scriptures* (New York: Penguin, 1959), 136.

5   Just as I mix the traditional Kuan Yin with contemporary life in the written vignettes, I also mix traditional art with present life in the illustrations I drew. Someone asked me if I was "appropriating" Kuan Yin (did I hear "misappropriating"?), but cultures have always adopted Kuan Yin with large changes (from

Indian male to Chinese female), and individuals within cultures have in turn modified their Kuan Yin for contemporary needs. For example, when women needed sons for validation in their society, they prayed to a "child-granting" Kuan Yin. But when women in Taiwan from the early nineteenth to the early twentieth centuries participated in a "marriage resistance movement," they gained financial independence as silk workers who lived in houses with one room dedicated to "independent" Kuan Yin. See Barbara E. Reed, "The Gender Symbolism of Kuan-yin Bodhisattva," in *Buddhism, Sexuality, and Gender*, ed. José Ignacio Cabezón (Albany: State University of New York Press, 1992), 169.

The Moon in the Water

Dug Up Kuan Yin

Someone has chiseled Kuan Yin on a slab of stone. As near as I can make out from the photo in a book, she sits on the ground on her island, holding a willow sprig in one hand and a water jar in the other. The outline of the full moon marks her off from rows of etched calligraphy, in two separate inscriptions. According to the translator, one Chinese worshipper in the eleventh century wrote that he had lost his father and was making this prayer stone for Kuan Yin. Much later, a magistrate in the seventeenth century recorded, closer to the artwork, that people lost track of the slab until a farmer dug it out of a field and gave the ridged and dirt-clogged stone to his daughter, to scrub clothes. Then (so goes the story) the washboard began to glow. . . .

In May 2001, I'm emptying out Dad's house in New Jersey, where he's lived for fifty years, and notifying his friends that he's planning to move to my apartment in Hawai'i in a month. The old house is the one I grew up in, so I have memories stashed here too, but for the moment, unwelcoming *stuff* overwhelms me: rows of lawnmower guts and chassis, unconnected, receipts from gas and electric bills going back to Methuselah. Upstairs, cast-off furniture huddles together, the very names fallen out of use: chiffonier, china closet, vanity, commode. My heart catches at the furniture Dad has built himself, incredibly beautiful, but too heavy and too many to ship to Honolulu. I convince cousins to lug away precious pieces, hoping that if I manage to visit them some day, I might find Dad's cobbler's bench, on which he incised a tree, or rediscover his clothes chest, making a new life for itself with some other child's mittens.

Dad's pals from the firehouse bring him a plaque. For their send-off, they roll up in style, clinging to the long hook-and-ladder truck. The neighbors must think the house is on fire. As a kid, I'd hear Dad get up in the night at the siren's summoning. I'd try to stay awake until he returned, safe. Recalling these vigils digs out the memory of his return vigils, at his small child's bedside: rubbing my back and waiting for me to fall asleep. Now the gray-haired firemen and the younger ones, who know Dad from quieter years as firehouse secretary, troop into the living room to read their etched plaque aloud: "in sincere appreciation. . . ." Standing at the screen door with his walker, the old volunteer watches them go. When these Kuan Yins pull away from the curb, tooting their horn, Dad laughs — the only time in a morose month.

Down cellar, I breathe cool mustiness and survey boxes, jars, drawers of nails, screws, bolts, and whatnots, plus a stack of unplayable 78-rpm phonograph records, homemade by Gram on a machine that spun out fragrant black hair and put Mom's songs in the grooves. I invite Aunt Verna to the cellar for souvenirs. She pokes at empty mason jars, formerly filled with Dad's red grape juice, transformed from blue grapes, and his cucumber pickle, whose turmeric painted the whole kitchen yellow. Suddenly Verna's eyes light up: "I've been looking for Mummum's doily stretcher!" She must have been looking a long time, as that grandmother died — let's see — forty-one years ago, when Dad brought the contraption home from his

The Moon in the Water

parents' dismantled cellar. He's been using it, unrecognized, to hang tools, until the pegged board glows back into an un-snarler of washed lace.

Pat, Dad's employee but also buddy, is devastated at his impending move to Honolulu. She has helped him since his bypass surgery in 1996 by cleaning up the house and rubbing his back; he helps her by repairing her vacuum cleaner and listening, probably one of the few to do so in her crowded day. Together they planted an unclaimed back field in collard greens and strawberries. "I ain't no young chippie," Pat sighs, but if they'd met a decade or so earlier, a few of the sparks crossing may have caught fire. He gives her Mummum's oak sideboard and the van, which he used to transport his electric cart to the grocery, when he could still drive. Now when Pat comes over to say good-bye, she cries, and Dad sinks more into himself.

Before packing his firehouse plaque, Dad is rereading its chiseled gold letters. When he comes to the lines "We wish you health and happiness in your new home in paradise," he frowns. "Do they think I'm dying?" I tell him the firemen are echoing marketers' jargon for tourists to a Pacific island. "I ain't going on vacation," he mutters.

I'm still sorting and tossing out *stuff*. Finally I've lured or begged or cajoled people to cart away all the tables and picture frames, and the house stands nearly bare. In the attic, I sweep up pins from the old sewing machine, ladybug bodies from summers past, and, inside the cedar closet, one red sassafras leaf. That sassafras tree disappeared years ago, cut down for reasons now lost. But here, in this empty space, lies a sassafras leaf found: still red, still glowing.

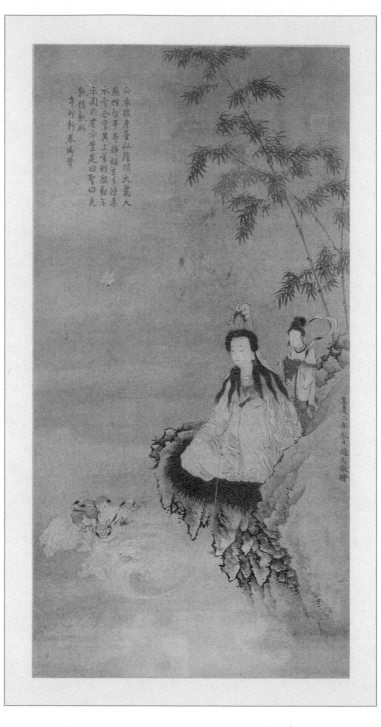

Pilgrim Gifts

This illustration, with a gold cast over the entire picture, shows Kuan Yin perched on a rock, with three bamboo stalks. A girl behind her and a boy on an opposite shore present some kind of undulating banners. Kuan Yin pours sustenance from her jar, and its delicate stream swells into the sea surge. The waves, the swirls of the drapery (blowing as if in a gale), and the squiggles of rock all follow the same pattern. Sometimes it's hard to tell rock from water.

Dad is putting together the recent past: "Somebody took me to the Philadelphia airport in a big car." "Yes, that was your niece Joy." "You two must have been in cahoots." "And you too, Dad. We didn't kidnap you!"

Somebody picks us up at Honolulu International Airport too. Mark, the first in a long line of Hawai'i friends who turn into helpers for Dad, rents a wheelchair and meets us at the gate. At home, Suzanne stops by with a jigsaw puzzle, whose picture of seashells—broken, for now—Dad drifts into piles. She also brings homemade chocolate-chip cookies, gone in a day. "Those were *good*," he pronounces, the most enthusiasm I've heard since he moved in.

Another friend, Lorna, hearing that Dad favors soft foods, arrives with a tin of custard powder and a quart of milk, then (already surpassing my capacities as a daughter) stirs at the stove for forty minutes. Cheryl offers a trip to the aquarium, hefting the heavy wheelchair into her trunk. Not one to give compliments face to face, Dad later praises her to me. He's glad to have seen the exhibits, but he also admires that "she didn't tarry" at any one fish. The most important thing is to keep one step ahead of looming tiredness.

When the wheelchair rental runs out, I decide to splurge on a lighter one, for chair-pushers less athletic than Cheryl. Joe drives to the shop, dissuades me from purple titanium ("It's not Marvin"), and slings a sensible "companionate chair" into the truck bed. But Dad is devastated at having no input whatsoever; he wants side wheels, so I go out questing again, and Joe slings around more chairs, small wheels, big wheels, till the Goldilocks traipsing from store to store is satisfied.

The bears are not satisfied. Now the bed is not right. Richard rigs up wood blocks to raise the foot of my old bed. (I've moved to a futon in the study.) Charlene sends muffins. When Dad's shoes won't fit his swollen feet, Deb finds him a pair of Velcroed, size-twelve slippers. (He calls them "slop-pers.") On her own initiative, my neighbor Nora, downstairs, begins lugging a few extra groceries for us: a half gallon of milk, or a hand of bananas. One day when we're tallying up, I ask Nora if she'll teach me to say "Water-Moon Kuan Yin" in Cantonese. "Kuan Yin" sounds like "Goon Yum." "Water-Moon" sounds like "soy yih-guong." Nora tells me that during the Cultural Revolution in China, she had to stand guard for her mom to —. Her English failing her here, Nora shakes her joined hands. After an initial impression of mom shaking the dice, I get the correct picture of her mother bowing joined hands to Goon Yum and defying the government prohibition

The Moon in the Water

against religion. Or maybe the first picture of gambling hits the mark too; those two women knew how to take risks.

When Nora's daughter Marty, age seven, stays here for a few hours, she encourages Dad to get out of bed and visit with us by doing her dog imitation: padding on all fours into his room, then yipping excitedly when he reaches for his walker. Dad smiles. He agrees to play "Go Fish" with the dog. "Do you have any Jacks?" she pipes. "Go fish." "Your turn," she keeps reminding him.

He's on a different shore, already. From his rock he accepts our paltry gifts, humors us, smiles. The rocks and the waves are blending together. Kuan Yin knows: Both are gold, both are flowing.

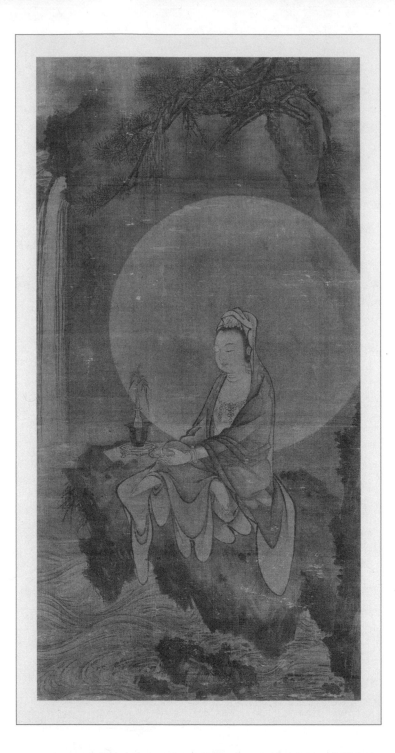

Water Pill

In this picture, Kuan Yin sits on an embankment. The
water has bitten out the underside, in chunks. Ink squiggles
swirl below. The whole overhanging bank will just let loose,
in one of these frames, in one big chunk.

On her tiny peninsula, Kuan Yin hooks her hands
around one knee. The artist has folded the other leg under
her, but the angle is wrong. That puffy foot looks stuck on,
upside down. Meanwhile, a scraggly willow stem sticks out
of a bottle on the ground next to her. The bottle appears
to be sitting inside a bowl, as if the artist couldn't decide
which would look better. So we get both, bottle and bowl:
largesse, on a pincushion.

A waterfall trickles down at the left of the picture.
An enormous moon backs Kuan Yin, with her head in its
center and the lower circumference sweeping along with her
arm as she calmly reaches out and clasps her knee. What's
that at the top of the frame? Pine needles. The moon hangs
below the pine branch, a moon where it's not supposed to
be.

Dad takes one furosemide every morning. The folks I
grew up with called such diuretics "water pill." The pill is to
make water, churn water, hint it to the body, like a waterfall
tinkling down. Make shishi for mama. The body won't. It's

hoarding its water, in the feet, in the ankles, where water shouldn't be stuffed. Water seeps to the lungs. Can he drown in those drops? The ankles puff out, a waxy, waxing moon, with little latticed hatchings, like pine needles.

The pill is to make water, get rid of water. But water makes us. We're supposed to be water. The liver is 70 percent water. The muscles are 75 percent water. Even the dry part of bone, no marrow, is 25 percent water. The brain, as Kuan Yin sits on her embankment, thinking, squishes along at 85 percent water. By contrast, water forms only 80 percent of the blood. Sodium ions and chloride ions float in the blood, the same as in the ocean, and make us and the ocean, the blood and the water as it laps past her embankment, both taste of salt.

The water pill will cure all. The pill looms as a pale, puffy moon, backing the person. Look to it! Phone call to physician's assistant: "His water pill doesn't seem to be working." "Elevate his feet." "He does elevate them." "Higher." Higher than pine branches. Assistant: "How much Lasix does he take?" "He doesn't take Lasix; he takes furosemide." Impatiently: "Furosemide *is* Lasix." Dummy. Oh and, fool, that's not a moon in the sky, framing Kuan Yin. Instead of sky, it's more water, a whole sheet of it, holding a reflection of the moon. The moon hangs under the pines, where it's supposed to be.

The Moon in the Water

The Moon in the Computer

> Observe all dharmas as illusions, flames, dreams,
> the moon in the water, echoes, flowers in the sky,
> images reflected in a mirror, shadows made by light,
> magical creations. . . .
> —*Great Prajñā-pāramitā Sūtra*

When I call the heart doctor's office to schedule an appointment for Dad, the secretary comes back to the phone to ask when he can make the trip from Hilo. "He's in Honolulu." "He's back from Hilo?" "He never went to Hilo." "But he lives in Hilo?" It takes us a moment to figure out that this doctor treats two men with the same name. The first folder plucked from the file cabinet offers a near look-alike, but not the real moon.

This particular appointment will enable a technician to check Dad's defibrillator, the mysterious box protruding from his upper chest like a deck of cards in a high pocket, a skin pocket. When we arrive, we sit, then get ushered from the waiting room to an inner sanctum, to further await the high priest. The representative for the company that manufactured the defibrillator finally shows up. He pores over the file, then looks baffled. At first I think that he has been handed the wrong folder, the one belonging to the reflector Dad, but no. It turns out that the secretary has invited a rep from the wrong company. The man standing there in his tucked-in aloha shirt comes from some pacemaker company, a near look-alike of what we want, but not the real moon.

The dauntless secretary decides to try to snare down a new moon, same day. Forty-five minutes later, the right rep appears, the one whose company has put its logo on the magical creation stashed between skin layers, two inches below Dad's collarbone. This rep grunts, goes straight to work. He sticks four moonlets onto Dad's arms and legs, clips a wire to each, and snaps open his laptop. After awkwardly compressing his girth toward the plug, he holds up a square that resembles a computer mouse, hovering over the look-alike square on Dad's chest.

I venture to interrupt the technician's mesmerized stare into the watery screen. "Dad's defibrillator put out two shocks about a month ago. They flipped him over!" "Mmmm," says the rep. Dad usually launches this recollection by asking, "Was I lying on the floor in the bathroom with my feet by the toilet and my head on that white threshold?" Now when I'm the one to bring up this event, he doesn't deign to regale this preoccupied stranger with any details.

(At the first shock, Dad let out a yell, which wakened me, and, at the second jolt, another yell, which brought me scurrying. I'd been home in New Jersey for six days, and with all the information I was trying to absorb at once, on his medications, his nebulizer, his tangled finances, his house sale, I had just that afternoon glanced over the pamphlet called "Your Defibrillator": "If your device puts out two or more shocks within five minutes, you should probably call an ambulance." Or was it five shocks in two minutes? No. Just call.

At least six rescue workers, men and women, crowded into the dim hallway, all unusually tall, muscular, poured into tight clothes, and laden with heavy equipment. But they had the Kuan Yin touch. Two policemen gently lifted my six-foot dad to a desk chair grabbed from the bedroom, then stood aside to let a medic check vital signs. Since Dad could breathe and talk and marvel that he'd been lying upside down, with his feet by the toilet and his head on that white threshold, he slipped clear of a trip to the hospital, that time.)

Abridging all that, I just tell the manufacturer's representative that the magical box gave Dad two shocks so strong they knocked him over. The rep goes on reading his screen. Finally he looks up and says, "The shocks were at 2 a.m.?" He adds a slight, respectful, interrogative lilt to his declarative sentence, but he needn't have cast any doubt. The real heart is floating there, on the screen's placid, gray, all-telling surface. The moon is in the water.

Waterfall ID

In one picture that I see in a journal, Kuan Yin observes from a rocky outcropping, bigger at the top than the bottom, like a saltshaker. (I mean, that's the shape of a saltshaker in use. Maybe she'll fall through the holes, in her porous rock seat, at any little seismic tap.) An aureole encircles the bodhisattva's head, and another aureole, outline of the moon, encircles her whole body. A waterfall, distant and skinny, sluices beside her.

Dad wants to know if his railroad pension has followed him from direct deposit in New Jersey to direct deposit in Hawai'i. "We can move the pension as soon as we open a bank account for you," I assure him. "I'll do it today."

"Does your dad have a picture ID?" asks the bank clerk. "He had one—on a driver's license, but he gave up driving. His reflexes are not as quick as they used to be, and he voluntarily threw away his license, so as not to endanger others," I burst out proudly, thinking of my friends' elderly parents bumping stubbornly over curbs. Good citizenship, however, reaps him no rewards in the bank's karmic system. "You'll need a state ID, with a picture." "I could bring him in, in person," I offer valiantly, calculating the distance pushing a wheelchair. But no, the real moon won't do, only its reflection, caught on a card.

In order to get a state ID (to get a bank account, to get the pension moved), we need Dad's birth certificate. I know I just saw this raggedy paper recently—I noted his birthplace, Titusville, New Jersey—when I sorted through his shoeboxes of papers. I plucked the birth certificate from among the receipts for purchases of lawnmowers and such and tossed it in a parcel to ship to Hawai'i. Altogether we sent eleven parcels. The parcel with the birth certificate has not arrived.

Kuan Yin is sitting on her outcropping, eating a banana. After listening to the distant waterfall, peeling down the banana, and chewing contentedly, she leans over her rock to toss the banana skin. Hey, there's another waterfall, below this rock level. How many waterfalls are there, and how high *is* this rock face?

"Is my pension going into direct deposit here?" Dad asks. "As soon as we open a bank account," I say, feigning confidence. "We can open your bank account as soon as we get your state ID, as soon as we get the box with your birth certificate."

Finally all the parcels from New Jersey show up: no birth certificate. "I just saw that Titusville line." Too bad; I've lost the birth certificate. In order to get the state ID (to get the bank account, to get the pension moved), we call New Jersey for a copy of Dad's birth certificate. A chatty recorded message assures me that I will have no trouble obtaining this document. If I pay by check through the mail, I can receive his new certificate in eight weeks. If I pay by credit card over the phone, however, I can have his copy, even two copies, within a week.

Kuan Yin leans over her rock. Wonder how far that banana peel wandered? Did it ride down the falls, having a good old time? Has it snagged on a venturesome tree branch, where it might be graciously feasting the ants? Or has it plunged on, to discover yet new waterfalls? The only problem is, I have no credit card. Nor does Dad. We are the last two holdouts in America, believing a better citizen does not buy on time. However, citizenship has not made it into the karmic code of the records department any more than the bank's. In order to get the birth certificate soon (to get the state ID, to get the bank account, to get the pension moved), our friend Cheryl has offered to let us use her credit card number. She and Dad sit assembling a jigsaw puzzle as I place the call to New Jersey.

"Maiden name of mother of person requesting birth certificate," the recording demands. "Unangst!" I inform the machine triumphantly. "Middle name of mother of person requesting birth certificate," the recording demands. I'm stumped. "Dad," I interrupt one puzzle for another, "do you know Mummum's middle name?" He's stumped. We apologize to the machine, which remains unperturbed, perhaps deviously. The machine then replays all my answers, so I can make any corrections. For the next

The Moon in the Water

ten minutes I listen to myself, including the exuberant "Unangst!" and the colloquy about the middle name.

Finally the copy of the birth certificate arrives. We take a taxi to the state ID office (to get the bank account, to get the pension moved). Because traveling by cab was more expensive than I liked, I call to inquire about the Handi-Van for future trips. "You come to Palama to get a picture ID." "We have a picture ID," I announce proudly, fondly recalling the completed quest to get a usable credit card, to get the birth certificate, to get the picture, to get the bank account, to get the pension moved. "Not the state photo ID. This is a photo ID, made by the state."

I look up at the waterfall and catch sight of a falling banana peel, yellow and lovely, which snags on some leaves from a branch, just meshing with a crescent moon.

No Moon

Kuan Yin is gazing out from her promontory. The water-battered sides look hacked and leave her on an overhang that juts over the bay. She rests her chin in her hand and her elbow on her knee. Kuan Yin keeps peering down to catch the reflection of the moon on the water, but no moon appears.

Frustrated by illness and exhaustion, Dad suddenly starts getting angry. Anger has never been part of my experience of him. Now he clumps into my room with his aluminum walker: "You didn't give me my medicine." Um, I did. "I used to be able to sleep until you took away my medicine." Uh —. The waves slice at the cliffs, the supports eroding, for several days. Finally Dad notices the undermining change: "I need an appointment with my Primary Care Physician. There's something wrong with me mind."

Me mind. Is this an Irish turn of phrase? The Irish playwright Samuel Beckett has his character Nagg, stuck in a trash can, beg his disdainful son Hamm, himself stuck in a wheelchair, for "me pap," "me sugar plum." Hamm bribes his old dad to listen to a pompous story by promising him a sugarplum. Once Nagg has endured the narration, Hamm reneges, with spiteful satisfaction, "There are no more sugarplums."

No sugarplums for me mind. I don't know where my family may have grafted any Irish forebears, but we did inherit Irish expressions. "I'll take the shillelagh to you," my parents used to warn—entirely in jest, as they never raised a hand or rod against me, not even the faintest smack. They just brandished the *word* shillelagh, because they liked the flow of it. Again sounding Irish, my mother would sigh, in moments of disgust, "Oh, Mother McCrea." Who Mother McCrea was and what she had to complain of, I couldn't tell you.

My mother, Madeline, savored words. One day she sat down and made a list of laments and curses, interjections and exasperations, starting with "Oh, Mother McCrea." The list grumbled on with "For Pete's sake," "Oh, for crying in a bucket," "Judas Priest" (all the consonants popping), "Hell's Bells," "Jumpin' Jehosaphat," "Oy vey," "Where in tarnation," and "Thunderation." The list sputtered out with "Shucks," "Shoot," and "Darn it," the constipated variants of "Shit" and "Damn." I could add the local Hawai'i version, "Oh, shoots," or the more juicily venomous "Shebai."

Dad could use a few good curses: "Dang nab it, these bowels." "Crikey, what if this bum leg gives out entirely?" "Those teeth had a harries of a time just with the raisins." (Usually "those teeth" bathe untaxed in their cup.) "Criminentlies, is that doctor's office at the *end* of this hall?" Though I have never once heard the F-word pass his lips, he might be considering deploying it at last, "Why am I so F-ing *tired*?"

Kuan Yin had better come up with some good blessings to do the real building, after the curses have fended off Bad Wind and cleared a space—if they can even do that much. Curses are the Special Forces of the palate, anathematizing any and all real or imagined foes for the sake of revenge, rather than justice, and hardly winning hearts and minds in the process. Kuan Yin would speak more to the point. May all your fungal toenails grow in clean. May the alveoli in your gummed-up lungs (the legacy of pneumonia) breathe open with joy. May your transition to spirit—when it comes to that—be painless and, yes, jolly. May your #@!#! daughter not give you too much grief while you're here, in the dark of the moon.

The Moon in the Water

Yankee Moon

One woodblock print shows Water-Moon Kuan Yin tucked
in a corner of rocks: a horizontal shelf to sit on, a lower rock
to rest her bare foot, and two flat outcroppings at either
side, just right to prop her elbows. The willow droops from
a cruet with a spout. An odd bird — it's upside down —
pinwheels above the waves. In the foreground, across the
water gap, two smaller figures hold out offerings from the
near shore. The circles around their heads exactly echo the
circle around Kuan Yin's. All three circles must be halos, or
at least hat brims: boaters, tilted back.

Dad is still disoriented in his new place. Up is down.
He puts his sandals on the wrong feet. He forgets basics.
After reminiscing about Mom one day, he asks, "Do you
remember Madeline? Or were you too young when she
died to remember her?" I'm shocked, as I was well into
adulthood at her death eighteen years ago. Of course I
remember her! But then memory turns out to be far from a
matter of course.

Dad is recollecting his old house. "I think 6 Fairfax has
been sold." "Well, it's on the market." "Somebody walked
off with my Yankee screwdriver." "Dad, that was your

nephew." "Jimmy'll never use that Yankee screwdriver." "Maybe not, but he'll value it. And it'll kick off stories: 'Remember when I used to visit Aunt Madeline and Uncle Marvin every summer? Marvin could make anything with those tools. He made a yo-yo on the lathe as big as his hand. . . .'" "Who took the yo-yo?" "Nobody took the yo-yo!" That yo-yo has been out of the picture for decades.

Sometimes Dad asks to sit outside his new building, on its tiny strip of lawn. He wears his denim hat because water pills make his skin intolerant to sunlight. One day when I fetch him, his hat is soaking wet. "It flew off." Even in a drought, drainage is so poor here that the twenty minutes of rain we've had in a month have left a small lake. And the trade winds are brisk. As I silently wonder about the miracles of hat retrieval from a wheelchair, he volunteers, "Some lady rescued it."

My friends Chip and Charlene come over to meet Dad. Charlene has brought homemade bread, "inside out," Dad says. She must have folded back the dough somehow, so it baked open, like a hat, a prelate's four-peaked concoction. Dad says, "I think 6 Fairfax has been sold." "Pretty soon." "Somebody walked off with my Yankee screwdriver." When Chip asks, "What did you build?" Dad perks up and talks a blue streak.

To distract Dad from the house sale, I take him to watch Japanese Bon dancing ("O-bon" in Japan). The

The Moon in the Water

Koganji Buddhist temple in Mānoa sits at the bottom of a deep hollow. After a friend has dropped us off, I gaze at the green Mānoa hills, but Dad eyes the long, steep driveway from a wheelchair perspective. Can his small daughter possibly push him back up that precipice? Can his arms that turned the lathe haul him up cliffs?

The Bon dancers are pinwheeling, clapping time with wooden sticks. An old man shuffles through the steps, holding a child. The toddler in the old man's arms grasps the sticks and claps them for him. More accurately, the toddler swings the sticks, wildly. The flailing sticks come nowhere near meeting, let alone keeping the rhythm. I let somebody walk off with his screwdriver.

The Bon dancers are now back-stepping some kind of samba-Bon. Dad is peering apprehensively at the long climb. I decide to abandon the zoris and corndogs and twirling fans and start our trek. I pounce on somebody with a cell phone. In his boater hat, he agrees to call a cab for us. Somebody else — another boater hat, nudged back on his sweating forehead — huffs and puffs to the top of the driveway, tugboating Dad's wheelchair. A teenage boy — same boater, next generation — dashes out to stop traffic so the cab driver can load the Bon revelers with wheelchair. "You're not Japanese!" the Filipino cabbie exclaims in astonishment, as we turn his slots for travelers upside down.

On the same day that Dad signs the papers to sell his

house at 6 Fairfax Drive, laboriously drawing his signature over and over, like a child's exercise of contrition, Chip brings Dad a gift. In a hurry to rescue his illegally parked car, he tips his straw hat as he leaves. Dad slowly unwraps the tissue paper. When he sees the new Yankee screwdriver, he laughs out loud.

Dad retells the Bon dancing only as, "Was I somewhere down in a pit?" I retell it as the boaters of strangers, the hats of friends.

Transferring the Willow

In one painting, Kuan Yin occupies a tiny island, with just enough room for four bamboo stalks behind her. Her right foot is tucked under the left knee, while the left foot hangs over the side of the island, to rest on a red lotus. In her right hand she holds a willow sprig; in her left, a vase, into which she is about to slip the fresh-cut branch.

To transfer Dad's medical insurance from New Jersey to Hawai'i, I call the Hawai'i Medical Service Association. An HMSA worker, Harriet, sends me six booklets to choose from, each fifty pages. Hazarding the "65C Plus" plan, I fill out the application, which asks for a copy of Dad's Medicare card. He says it's in his wallet. I unfold the dilapidated leather and find a picture of Mom from half a century ago, wearing bobby socks and a tight sweater; a picture of me as a baby, wearing nothing; ah, a card with "Horizon Medicare Blue" blazoned along the border. I saunter to the copy center, tape the image to the form, and pop the envelope into the mailbox.

Kuan Yin sits at ease, her foot still propped on a glowing red lotus. Other lotuses, red and bluish purple, poke up behind her, the same size whether in front or back of the island. Under the bamboo, some unidentified spheres stand spitted like shish kebabs. The outline of the tiny island forms the bottom half of a circle, which continues above Kuan Yin's torso and head, a kind of spotlight, with only her foot dangling beyond her private bubble. The willow in her right hand hasn't moved any closer to the vase in her left.

Weeks later, HMSA sends back my application, rejected: "The card you submitted is not a Medicare card." I call Harriet. "Dad's card says Medicare." "It's not Medicare." "It says Horizon Medicare Blue." "Blue is different. A real Medicare card has a red stripe." Harriet pauses. "Is your father an American citizen?" "Yes." "Is he past sixty-five?" "He's seventy-eight." "Then he has a Medicare card." Wrong lotus.

Kuan Yin sits on her island. Her turf offers just enough room for four bamboo stalks, creaking in the breeze. The lake with the red and blue lotuses completely encircles her bubble, and the expanse of water has its own horizon at the top of the painting. In her left hand she holds her vase of water. In her right hand she trails the willow branch, looking bedraggled.

"Is this the Railroad Retirement Board? I'm calling about my dad's Medicare card." "Retirement number, please." "_____." "Ah, he has Horizon Medicare Blue."

The Moon in the Water

"I know that. It's the wrong lotus." "Well, try calling Horizon." "Dawn speaking." No, Dawn has never seen a lotus. She suggests I call the Railroad Retirement Medicare Office. "Ted here." Ted has no record of Dad's Medicare number. "Try our old Medicare office." I repeat my mantra: Medicare, Medicare. The twelfth person I talk to gives me a phone number I recognize as that of the first person I called. Kuan Yin's bubble is round, the lake is round, and we're up to the thirteenth moon.

On her island in the lotus lake, Kuan Yin sits relaxed. She sports jewelry on both wrists, both ears, her neck. She's wearing harem pants, as her right ankle rests fetchingly under her left leg. I could do with a pair of harem pants. I could do with a harem, some nice women to talk to, a pasha to cuddle up to, now and then. In her right hand, she flicks the willow branch. In her left hand, she's tilting the water vase. Has she given up transferring the willow?

After six more weeks, I manage to extract from the Railroad Retirement Board a Medicare card with a glowing red stripe. Harriet has insisted so religiously on this stripe that I ask the worker at the copy center, Clifford, to duplicate it in color. He looks at me suspiciously. "We can't do that," he says, as I try to stamp the moon in the water. So I tape the black-and-white version of the red-striped card onto the rejected application and hike the envelope to the mailbox.

Kuan Yin's willow hasn't moved any closer to the water in the vase. I know I've seen prints of that willow *in* the vase, on the ground next to her, as she sits on her embankment. But wait. Here it says the willow and the container were originally separate, unrelated. The willow isn't just sitting there, static decoration. Instead, it's busy whisking away disease (and, presumably, warding off the bills of illness). What I thought was a vase is a bottle, pouring the water of Contentment Anywhere.

Harriet calls: "You sent the page that says 'patient's copy.' We need the one that says 'HMSA copy.'" "They're identical," I say. "But you sent the page that says 'patient's copy,'" Harriet reminds me. "*Cross out* 'patient's copy,'" I venture to suggest, "and *write in* 'HMSA copy.' Everything else is identical." "No," says Harriet, "you'll have to file a new application." Well, I can do that. After all, I'm wearing my harem pants, chatting with Harriet and Dawn and Clifford, eating my shish kebabs, and touch-toning innumerable numbers on my lotus pad, connected to the circling worlds.

Willy Moon

Kuan Yin is sitting on a rock at the edge of the water, one
ankle resting on the other knee. This time she surprises
me by holding a baby, whose feet are standing shakily on
her bent leg. This Child-Giving Kuan Yin is later than
the Water-Moon Kuan Yin but still draws on the earlier
conventions: same willow in a jar, same surrounding water-
swirls. Oh, and her raised foot again looks upside down:
same string of hacks copying a master's pattern but still not
quite getting the hang of the job. A bird swoops low, eyeing
the willow, as the baby reaches up gleefully.

Dad is dragging around on his swollen feet, worn out,
lonesome for his old home, uncomplaining. I can't think
of anything to say. I keep getting, then losing, the hang
of this job. Meanwhile, Willy Lump-Lump is lounging
in his blue-and-white striped nightshirt on the bureau in
the room where Dad is now living. This seven-inch rag
doll, battered and begrimed, has survived the years since
Dad made him for me at the sewing machine. I must have
been about six then, for my eyes just matched the level of
Dad's big work hands, guiding the cloth under the machine
needle, pounding away. Of course, sometimes a sewing
machine needle races ahead of even the best work hands,

and Will emerged from the creative fit with one small foot and one big foot, one small arm, one big arm, plus a frankly hydrocephalic head.

Yes, I did have the word hydrocephalic in my vocabulary as a child, but not until three years later, when I stayed in the hospital for a week by myself—I mean, without my parents—to have my own oddly formed feet operated on. I was by myself, but whenever I managed to turn my gaze away from the large, shocking absence of my parents, I noticed that I was far from alone, for I met Norman, with a hernia; Julie, with leukemia; and my nameless roommate, a silent baby with hydrocephalus. I at least observed, if I did not properly meet, this child with water on the brain, water making his head moon. I remember that the baby's head bulged out, like Will's after his turn around the sewing machine. Kuan Yin's breast, as the baby leans against her, picks up the pulse from that bounding brain, unaccommodated by usual bodies.

Will's brain was fine, despite his head size, so Dad hand-stitched him wistful dashes for each eye and a faint smile, to indicate that the lumpy lad was unfazed by mismatched left and right sides. Now, many years later, Will "speaks" as I move him over to Dad's bed. "What do they mean, 'Elevate your feet, elevate your feet?'" Will complains, holding up his big, water-retaining foot. "Do they mean I should stand on my head?" Will flips over sarcastically, to illustrate the blithe mandates of doctors. Dad laughs. Ah, a toe drawn right.

Dad is remembering: "I liked it when he had a red heart." A portrait of Will with a red heart had winged its way to the hospital in a get-well letter when Dad received his implanted defibrillator, six months ago. Dad ponders, "Does he have a red heart now?" and takes the liberty of checking under Will's frayed nightshirt. "Well," I prevaricate, "he insisted I draw a red heart on his portrait in a letter to you at the hospital." Dad is enormously pleased. "I can't believe I was just messin' around at the sewing machine one day, poked the cloth inside out and stuffed it, and he's still in the, in the *talk*. You never know what'll turn out to be important." "'Course I'm important. Just 'cause I'm bald now," I ventriloquize for Will. Dad muses for a while: "He was never not bald."

In the get-well letter, which I found still afloat on Dad's card table in New Jersey eight weeks after posting, the words along the left side of that distinctive silhouette — one big foot, hydrocephalic head — reported that Will had called me from the bureau drawer, asking a favor. "Sure, Will. What is it?" "Would you write to Marvin and tell him that I was just sitting here thinking, when it occurred to me that if it weren't for him, I would have remained a shapeless wad of cloth!" Kuan Yin verifies the moon in the sky by gazing elsewhere, down in the water.

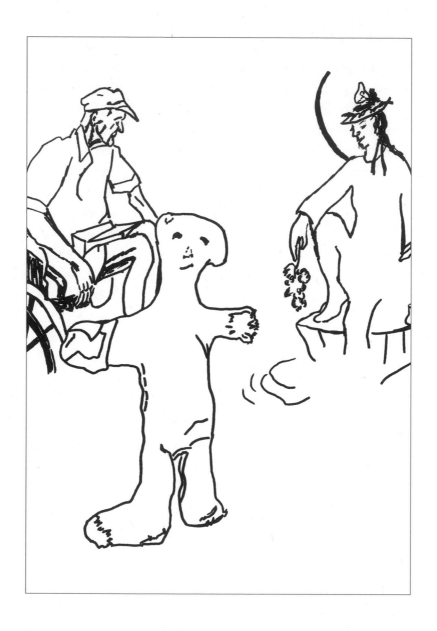

Artsy Crappy Moon

The exhibit of "Esoteric Buddhism" at the museum includes a "Kuan Yin with Willow" of the water-moon type. The artist has painted her with one knee drawn up and one foot on her rock seat. The willow—for healing, says the blurb on the wall—must be standing in that vase at the grimy edge of the scroll, though the vase looks empty to me.

The neighbor from the next apartment, Mrs. K., stops by with a piece of strawberry shortcake "for papa-san." "If you want to know what ails me," he says to her, devouring the cake so fast you'd think I never feed him, "I'm homesick." "Oh, I missed Japan too. When I first moved here, I would look out at the Mānoa hills and think back to the hills at home. I cried every day. Is that how you feel?" "Prett' near."

Mrs. K. suggests the Mō'ili'ili Senior Center, so, in an effort to cure Dad's doldrums after his move to Honolulu, I bring a pamphlet from the senior center to the breakfast table. Actually, the list of activities is not promising. Aerobics, tai chi, and square dancing assume some pretty sprightly elders. Scrabble? Not this creative speller. "Darts?" "You're kidding," he says, mashing up a banana for his cereal.

He starts reading my bread wrapper instead of the seniors' pamphlet: "Your chance to enter and win $1,000,000!" He declines the offer. "I don't want a million dollars. Everybody'd be pesterin' you." It's true he's not greedy. He let a neighbor, fresh from a messy divorce with no funds, live with her daughter in his cellar for a year. If he had hangers-on as a poor man, think of his petitioners as a millionaire. And "pesterin'" would soon weigh on this loner. On the other hand, as the memory of the rent-free tenants also attests, he's not a complete loner. I resuscitate the ad from the senior center.

"How about feather-lei making?" I suggest, looking around my apartment at the evidence of skill with his hands. Long ago he gave me bookends from slices of tree limbs, sanded and glued to a metal base. To one wall, he has nailed a two-foot bookshelf, one quarter of a cherry log with the bark still left on the curve. He also sent that little footstool, in separate pieces, trusting to my shaky ability to rematerialize it whole. (He had drilled the first hole in the wrong place but compensated for the miscalculation by drilling a second hole and declaring, in pencil, next to the first: "Not a hole." This clear hole which is not a hole has always somehow pleased me.) To bolster my case for his inventions, I point out the rainbows scattering from a prism, which he suspended from the open louvers with an elaborate arrangement of wire and string: "Some clever guy I know rigged that up." He smiles. He agrees to go to the senior center to try seed craft.

The Moon in the Water

The Water-Moon Kuan Yin at the museum is wearing some kind of gauzy, intermittently transparent drapery, exquisitely worked with hexagons in green and red and gold. Whoever wove such cloth must have put in hundreds of hours, and painting the wearer on a silk scroll from a model must have exhausted the artist in turn. A coating of soot has seeped into the silk so that the green and gold and red scarcely retain a hint of their former selves.

Before Dad has a chance to change his mind about joining a group, I leave the breakfast dishes and push him in his wheelchair to the Mōʻiliʻili Senior Center. Despite the name on the gate, a horde of juniors swarms out of Summer Arts and Crafts. Though they part like the Red Sea, Dad hunkers down as doubtfully as Pharaoh in his chariot. Finally the children peter out and we roll onward, to seed craft. A roomful of elderly Japanese women looks up in consternation as this large *haole* man with small attendant barrels into their midst. "May he join your group?" I ask. After a long moment, one seed polisher admits sadly that their teacher has gone on vacation for the summer and they are merely filing the seeds. She motions us on to feather leis next door. "May he join your group?" After the familiar pause among the exclusively female clientele, one worker holds out a hatband to show us her elegant stitches. "We're *sewing* the feathers," she explains, emphasizing skill and looking skeptically at Dad. "He sews!" I announce triumphantly. As a brakeman, Dad used to sew patches on his work pants. Of course, he did match red patches with green thread on blue denim, but he fastened the cloth securely enough. And he sewed Will, who is still part of our household. "Just because I'm forty-five years old," Will was blustering only yesterday, calculating his age from my six years at his birth, "don't go thinking I'm ready for the shelf yet!" Dad had looked at his still-speaking handiwork and then at his daughter: "I believe you've gotten more pleasure out of that toy than any store-boughten doll-babies!" "Store-boughten doll-babies!" Will had scoffed. "There's no comparison!" Here at the Mō'ili'ili Senior Center, I tell Will he'd better pipe down (hey, has he tagged along?) and not go strutting his stuff (or stuffing) before the ladies.

Dad decides: "I ain't stickin' feathers on no ties." We roll out. He is craning his neck to admire the flowering trees. I stop pushing. Here are the golden shower trees, drooping down, huge yellow clusters with pink blushes guarding the flowers still to bloom. The gauzy Kuan Yin is sitting quietly, holding a feather that dropped in her lap from some fast-flying sea bird, or, no, behind the soot, she's waving the branch of some graceful tree.

The Moon in the Water

Moon Body

Kuan Yin has moseyed off to a rocky niche in a grotto, charcoal gray, next to cliffs plunging toward water. The pines shoot up vigorously, towering over a paper-paneled hut, like a bathhouse. The tumbling clouds are also brewing up a charcoal gray, dunking the moon in and out of wind and water. As Kuan Yin gazes at the moon-wisps, her pale orange shawl swings open negligently, on the way to the bath.

Dad is getting washed. Not so confident any more at climbing into the tub, even with rails and a shower chair in his own niche, he lowers himself to the closed toilet seat to let me help him bathe. I hand him the purple sponge, vivid when wet, and remind him, "That's soaped; watch your eyes" or "Dry that arm." He pauses at the conundrum of watching his own eyes. Each session he laughs at my same feeble jokes, as I scrub past the "chicken coop," the ripple of bone left under his skin from bypass surgery. Every time I praise, "Look at these beautiful hands," he obediently turns over his gentle work hands and gazes at them wonderingly.

It's Mom who taught us this ease with bodies. The family never displayed casual nudity, but they clearly knew the body made joy, and if it had pain instead, or needed help, you could surely squeeze out some good juice somewhere. Back when Mom had a hernia operation, Dad would slip to her room to help change bandages, and she would ad-lib jokes, though the nine-inch cut on her belly refused to heal up. Her diabetes-stunned tissues left an inch-wide gap, plunging to a V, wet like a spring-fed grotto. Still, I'd hear the two of them, sequestered, giggling like teenagers.

Now at home in Honolulu, my role is to wash unreachable spots and some available ones, when he loses interest. Soaping his hands, I note the hint of blue tinting the skin between thumb and finger and roping his arms, from thinned blood seeping: pooling, greening. When I hand him the sponge and prompt, "This is for your genitals," he makes the foreskin slip up and down like a loose sock. He stands to wash his bottom. Weird, this American culture, to make an insult of flashing the moon.

Then, as part of the ritual, when I ask him to hang the towel on its rack, which is taller than I am, he always chuckles at being able to help *me*. In fact, I discovered recently that this goal is his whole reason for staying. Tucking him in one night, I asked if he wanted to turn on his other side, to give a developing bedsore a rest. No, he prefers to lie permanently on his deaf left ear, to leave his right ear listening, even while asleep: "in case you call for help."

Kuan Yin Prescription

Ch'an monks during the T'ang dynasty liked to play
with possible meanings for Kuan Yin's water-moon
imagery. Ch'an teacher Shih-t'ou Hsi-ch'ien (700–790
c.e.) emphasized permanence within impermanence: "Are
there birth and death for the moon in the water or the
reflection in the mirror? You must know that you already
have everything within you." As he watched the flitting and
fading of lychees, chances, honors, friends, Shih-t'ou must
have been striving not to fret or grieve — but not to give up
on the kaleidoscope either. He kept dashing out into the
world to view its slippery, dazzling patterns, perplexing as
they were. Appreciating the alleyway as well as the temple,
the teacher judged that "ultimate truth" could be "possessed
by the worldly as well as the sages." He concluded:
"Enlightenment and vexations are the same in essence,
although they differ in name."

Dad is doing a jigsaw puzzle. He has carefully turned
over all the pieces for the Springbok scene of seashells
on a beach. I used to shun jigsaw puzzles as boring, but
now I poke around in the colors to keep Dad company. It

occurs to me that my usual activities of research and writing don't differ all that much from his passion for puzzles: scanning a mass of jumbled material, searching for patterns, testing if this fits that. We must share a common gene for "puzzler," with a long attention span.

Dad has just taken his morning pills: Coreg, Zestril, aspirin, potassium, vitamin. The pharmacist's printout warns him not to lie down for thirty minutes after swallowing the potassium, so it doesn't settle in the esophagus. At the same time, a couple of the other bottles announce, in sticky labels with a tiny picture of a droopy eyelid, that "this product may cause drowsiness." The lure of the jigsaw is keeping Dad awake till the potassium slides down. Dutifully upright at his table, he is fingering and grouping the fragments of calico scallops, volutes, starfish, stones.

Drowsiness wins. Dad goes back to bed, I to my desk, to fill out another discount application, urged by the pharmacist. We already sent in one form, for an Orange Card from the manufacturer of a heart pill: "Draw all the letters of your name, address, and situation in separate rectangles and wait six weeks." Twelve cardless weeks have passed. So now we give up on the Orange Card and apply for something called Good Life.

"When you take potassium," cautions the

pharmacist's blurb, "tell your doctor if you experience breathing trouble, chest pain, an irregular heartbeat, dark or tarry stools, confusion, tingling of the hands or feet, or stomach pain. If you notice other effects not listed above, contact your doctor or pharmacist." Ah, here's the part about the Good Life: "To increase your potassium, you can also eat bananas, citrus fruits, avocados, prunes," though the instructions don't specify whether the prunes will counter or abet the dark and tarry poop.

After his nap, Dad wakes up with his recurrent conviction that something has fallen from the bed. "Hey, Kathy? I had a tomato, but—" "You had a tomato?" "Yeah. It got away from me." "You mean a mango? We have mangoes." "No, a tomato. I think it rolled under the bed." "It must have been a dream. Here, I'll look under the bed for you." "Oh. I thought I had a tomato. But why would I have a tomato in bed?" "The tomato wasn't in bed! *You're* in bed. The tomato is in your noggin." "Well, better there than making a spot on your carpet."

On the way out to the puzzle, in the props of the walker, he almost loses his balance: "Did you see me do that little dipsy?" "Mmmm." He manages to move to the chair and begins shifting his puzzle pieces again. He disentangles bits of a yellow starfish from a silvery-mauve one blending with the shallow water, which promises to extend into a rich blue across the whole right-hand corner. I interrupt to ask if he'll peel off a sock so I can inspect his feet. The heart doctor solved the problem of Dad's water retention by directing: "You'll have to be his kidney! You gauge how swollen his feet are, and you decide the dose for furosemide." If I ask Dad how puffy his feet feel, he joshes, "I don't have a micrometer." I hand him two tablets, and he goes back to corralling cephalopods across the table.

For water pills, Dad takes a blue booster, Zaroxolyn, along with the white furosemide; any change in dosage has to be checked now and then with a blood test, to see that the potassium is still balanced. In trying to match the little white tablets against puffiness, we discover that less is more. Too many jade the body. But if we back off, the body resumes its water-filtering task, with just a tap from the pills to remind it what to do. In this Tao of water-pill dosing, we trace the spaces as well as the juttings.

As Dad puts the finishing shapes into his jigsaw shoreline, he notices that the colored paper has peeled away from a lobe here, a hook there. I fetch the Elmer's glue, so he can dab a few flecks back to a sundial shell, a seaweed back to its sand. He patiently holds a thumb and finger against a pictured snail shell reared up from its cardboard base. The cardboard itself builds up from separate sheets of coarse paper; some places, the layers have all come apart, ruffling the round lobe into a tiny fan. Dad applies his glue to the world's ephemera, soothing down a nervous white squiggle on blue paper at the edge of the picture. That squiggle is nothing but the print of a photo of a sun-dapple, on a passing wave. Or the glint is Kuan Yin's moon-dapple, moving fast, over the water.

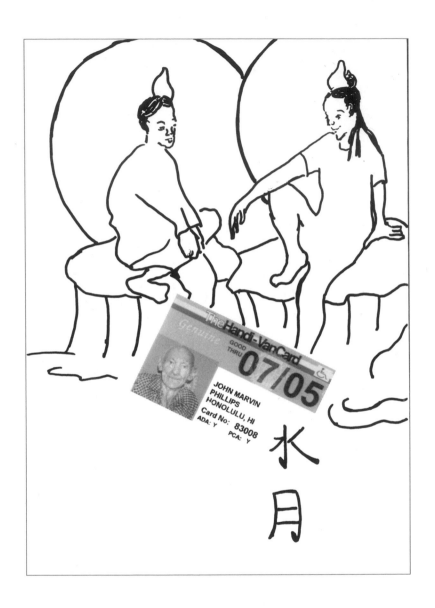

Riding the Tides in the Handi-Van

Around the edges of a tenth-century poster, called "Kuan Yin Appears in Twenty-Four Manifestations," little pictures crowd together in squares, like the path on a Monopoly board. In city center, instead of stacks of penalty cards, a garish Kuan Yin towers up through all the remaining space, eleven-headed, many armed, with multiple armbands: a fancy traffic cop. Most of the border pictures show nonhuman "manifestations": stubby plants, birds, an elephant. Two lone humans at the edge, tiny Water-Moon Kuan Yins, preside modestly at the top two corners, backed by full moons. One of these figures rests with her hands clasping her knee, on a cupcake-shaped island, gazing right. The other perches on a second cupcake, arm draped over a drawn-up knee. This Water-Moon Kuan Yin gazes left, waiting for her return ride, home.

Dad and I sit on the ledge of the potted plants at the bottom of our high-rise, watching for the Handi-Van. It's ten minutes before nine. Our doctor's appointment, a twenty-minute trip downtown by ordinary car, is at ten-thirty. The van is supposed to arrive in a "window," a forty-minute stretch within which, by a roll of the dice of red lights, traffic congestion, and alacrity of previous passengers, the wheels of the vehicle will finally halt at our very own doorstep. Meanwhile, Dad decides that the gray dove with powder-blue eye shadow, strutting in front of him and cooing lustily, is announcing, "I'm a bird, I'm a bird." Dad says maybe a human has taught the dove to speak, the way some pranksters teach parrots to do their swearing for them.

The blue-and-white van chugs around the corner, nearly as loud as the trash truck. Fishing for Dad's two-dollar fare and ID card, which authorizes me as PCA (Personal Care Attendant), I notice that tilting the card makes an iridescent circle appear over Dad's face: hey, a moon ring. Meanwhile, Dad is gliding lazily to the curb with his walker. The driver has lumbered around to lower the lift, but Dad ignores it and maneuvers himself and the walker up the steps. Somehow, with my slight bone deformity, I can't make these steps; the flimsy spokes for closing the door block my leaning spots. Anyway, I take the lift, as if I were the Handi-Van designee. These little laminated cards announcing identity sometimes deal lines at random.

After the driver stows the lift, clambers aboard, and turns into traffic, she starts popping sunflower seeds.

The Moon in the Water

Letting one hand do the steering, she swipes a seed from a bag clipped to the dash, chews, spits out the shell, deposits it in a box on the seat, and wipes her hand on a cloth. "I eat like a bird," she announces. Mom used to mutter skeptically at such demurrals, "Yeah, birds eat several times their own weight."

A passenger with a claw-footed walker toils aboard at Daiei Market. After she has laboriously settled into the seat in front of me, I ask if she would like to have her seatbelt, which is fastened inaccessibly behind her chair. When she doesn't reply, either because she doesn't hear, speaks another language, or has wearied of officious strangers, I unsnap the belt and offer an end around her side, but this is obviously a woman who scorns all restraint.

The van veers off into Mānoa Valley. Do not pass go; do not collect two hundred dollars. Whizzing past the Safeway, the Handi-Van squeezes into a maze of lanes and then into a bricked cul-de-sac, with red anthuriums flourishing lustily. Dad is craning forward to see the sights. Although the pamphlet of Handi-Van instructions forbids radios to passengers, the rule apparently exempts drivers. Unctuously coating all corners of the van, the voice of the president is announcing a new war. Towers come down, and hovels fly up. An elderly passenger thrashes forward through the anthuriums. "Slow down, slow down," a tottering companion cautions, to no effect.

"P O B Two!" the driver sings out. Dad's doctor holds court at Physicians' Office Building Two, as expensive to land on as Boardwalk with hotel; across the street sits an identical physicians' warren, Park Place with hotel. Dad negotiates the steps as the van belches exhaust. "It's my birthday!" the driver announces. Dad doesn't respond, either because he doesn't hear or can't tell how to stall her aging any more than his own. Once past the automated doors, he is already tiring. We spy an old-fashioned wheelchair, high and clunky, like the one in photographs of Mom as a child in Shriners' Hospital, where doctors kept her an incomprehensible seven months, instead of letting her recover better at home from orthopedic surgery. (Mom, the first in the family to have something like my odd bones, was told they weren't transmissible. Ha.) Dad lowers his six-foot height into the relic and lets his elbows, knees, and folded walker poke out like pick-up sticks.

With Dad now wearing a purple chiffon armband where a technician drew blood, we hurry down to the lobby and unfold Dad and his paraphernalia from the dilapidated chair. Our return trip was scheduled for

The Moon in the Water

noon; we've missed our van by five minutes. Other vans keep turning into POB One, across the street. A man on a bench rejoices that the Handi-Van has brought him all the way from Kapolei; another escort going back in that direction is due "in a couple of hours." Opposite this patient traveler, Dad is resting with his hands clasped around his knee. The full moon backs each of them separately, the same month, or a different one. Blue-and-white Handi-Vans keep turning the corner, like the waves.

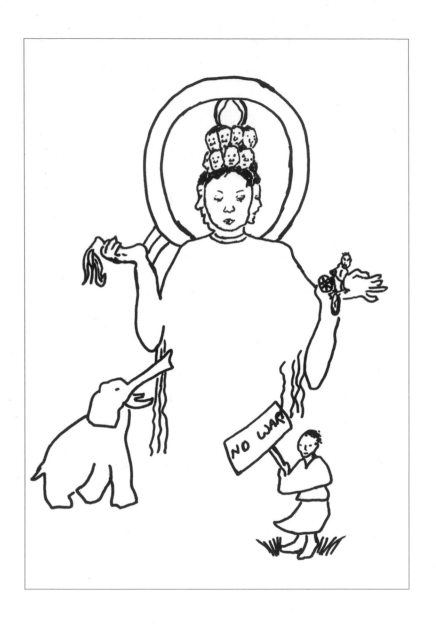

Peace Moon

In this same print, whose full title is "Kuan Yin Appears in Twenty-Four Manifestations in Response [to Prayers]," Water-Moon Kuan Yin occupies only two tiny rectangles. Back in the tenth century, Emperor Ch'ien Shu silk-screened twenty thousand copies of this sheet of multiple Kuan Yins. In the top corners, Water-Moon Kuan Yin's three-quarter left and three-quarter right profiles command the narrowest of crumbly islands. The water rushes threateningly around her, while the moon—repeatedly—circles her perch.

Dad has been napping, but he wakes up enough to help make a sign for the peace vigil. He cuts the poster board while I rummage for fat pens in black and pink. As I color in "No More Victims," vertically, like calligraphy, Dad spreads the glue on a flat stick, then holds the stick firmly to the back of the sign. His handiwork will be joining the protest against the bombing of Afghanistan, after the suicide hijackers crumpled the towers. Their fireball seared itself over and over into the collective psyche through television screens, but the Afghani houses crumble up with less fanfare.

Among Emperor Ch'ien Shu's silk-screened Kuan Yins, only two out of twenty-four manifestations even appear as human: those tiny, moon-gazing Kuan Yins at the margins. In the other squares, Kuan Yin squirrels herself away in nonhuman forms: "the fourth is the manifestation as auspicious grass, the fifth is the manifestation as a golden drum, the sixth is the manifestation as the hand of the Buddha . . . the tenth is the manifestation as a golden elephant." In the center of the print, the tall, many-headed Kuan Yin looks every which way. Rumor has it that one face laughs, but that rollicking grin doesn't show up from this angle.

On the grassy plot near the Honolulu Federal Building, the scarlet poinciana blossoms drift down and the peace vigilers straggle together. The signs say, "Our cry of grief is not a cry for war" and "Justice, not retaliation." One white-haired woman trudges over the grass with an American flag and a placard, "Peace is patriotic." Another protester waves the Hawaiian flag. A young man, black hair spiked green, stands at one corner of a painted banner, unfurling "There's no glory in slaughtering third-world countries." The Quaker, the revolutionary, and the couple with toddler hold up long, flimsy ti leaves, alternating with signs. When "Honk for Peace" pleas dot the lineup, drivers in the four lanes, slowing to the light, hearten us with elephant trumpetings.

As her way of commemorating the crumbling towers, my cousin has asked for the particulars of Dad's military service in World War II, to hang a plaque to the brothers'

The Moon in the Water

old "heroism." When I approach Dad, he waves aside the heroism; I know he does not gild those months in the Philippines. He especially dislikes the media's misuse of remembrance as a goad to supposed replays. If you ask Dad why the United States fought in Vietnam, the Persian Gulf, and now Afghanistan, he'll spit back his explanation, "Money!" During the earlier Gulf War, he urged, "Why aren't those college kids out protesting?"

At the Honolulu peace vigil, where I carry Dad's sign, some young men are unloading drums from a station wagon. They lug them onto the grass, patter uncertainly, then begin to play in dialogue, appreciating each other's improvisations and building on them. Signs proclaiming "Violence breeds violence" and "Jobs, not bombs" sprout at curbside. A man who has painted his face and arms green and wrapped himself in a green cloth sashays by in an elaborately flowered *haku* lei. I chalk up a Manifestation in Response. Another Manifestation (harder to see how this one is also a teacher) lurches his bicycle threateningly among the sign-holders, heckling us with his fluid pronouns: "They'll fuck you the way you fuck us."

Meanwhile, the scarlet poinciana are drifting down, on auspicious grass.

Moon Passing through Cloud

In a commemorative painting of one soul's passing, a central Water-Moon Kuan Yin sits on the ground, knee drawn up. The moon arcs around the calm figure, the bamboo flourish, and the large willow in its jar intersects the moon. In the lower left corner of this twelfth-century composition, the tiny dead man is standing, wearing his best blue robes. A stretch of water separates the mourners from the teacher and from the dead man. At the upper right, a boy—representing the dead man new in spirit— reaches down exuberantly, toward Kuan Yin's willow.

We get word that Dad's brother has died. Because Dad is too far away to go to the funeral, we decide to mark Elbert's passing here. My friend Cheryl, who adds her presence to our puny number of celebrants, helps scout the neighborhood for a body of water. We find a stream sliding under King Street, but the site is too noisy for a ceremony, so we spy out the rails for the stream's reemergence. From Kapiolani Boulevard, a vista opens out all the way to a blue hill, with the water ruffling over brown stones. I didn't even know this peaceful spot stood here, so close to home.

We test out possible wheelchair routes and return to fetch Dad. Cheryl has brought red hibiscus, white frangipani, red and white bleeding heart. Dad carries the box of our offerings and a camera on his lap as Cheryl pushes the chair. The sun makes us sweat and the few remaining unscooped curbs trip us up, but it feels right to be making a trek.

Dad is pleased to see the stream glittering ahead, between steep banks of purple bougainvillea. I read a short statement, shouting actually, so Dad can hear, but addressing Elbert:

> Uncle Elbert, we have here beautiful things: flower petals and blue eggshell. They are as fragile as the body, but they also float free as your spirit.
>
> Elbert, we hope you won't laugh when you see we have included also a dog-shaped animal cracker. It symbolizes the companionship you gave and the brotherly, fellow feeling we send along with you. May your spirit be light and joyous!

Dad tosses the red hibiscus. I snap photos of the stream, the tossing. From the rail, we can see the eggshell bobbing, as a java-rice bird on a low branch hopefully eyes the blue speck. The animal cracker dances jauntily, spins through an S-shaped eddy, and rests in the shallows. In the pictures, the red hibiscus glows. Even the animal cracker, a tiny dot, winks back at the camera.

Blue Moon

In this same painting of a soul's passing, Water-Moon
Kuan Yin sits relaxed on the ground, knee drawn up. In the
lower left corner, the tiny dead man is standing modestly,
wearing his best blue robes. At the upper right, his much-
rejuvenated self reaches out exuberantly. In the lower right
corner, across a stretch of water separating the mourners,
his loved ones play music, dance at the funeral.

I talk to Elbert's daughter on the phone to see how
the other mourners across the water have fared at the
graveside in Pennsylvania. She tells me about Elbert's
last week in the hospital. A small infection turned into
septicemia for this eighty-one-year-old, as his system
seemed to decide, "Enough a'ready." His hands along the
hospital sheets looked light blue. A nurse explained, "His
body is conserving energy for heart and lungs, letting limbs
go." Within a few days, Elbert's hands turned deep blue.
Finally, says Martha, his hands were the dark purple of
eggplant.

"Did I hear that George died?" Dad asks. "Elbert.
Elbert died last week. George died about ten years ago."
Dad shakes his head and laughs, at the antics of a memory

that somersaults facts over feelings. "I need a new memory."
He unbuttons two shirt buttons and delicately taps his
defibrillator. "Here's me new heart. It has a memory." I look
puzzled. "It remembered the shocks were at 2 a.m.," he
reminds me.

What would we program into a new memory box on
Dad's chest? We could put in that Elbert helped out when
Dad had surgery in 1996. My first hint of Dad's operation
came from his absence at the Philadelphia airport after my
routine flight from Honolulu. When I called home, Elbert
unexpectedly answered: "You know them things in your
legs? Well, they took four of 'em, *four* of 'em, and put 'em in
his *heart*!" "Heart" was the last word in the sentence. Good
thing I could dredge up miscellaneous information, that
surgeons pluck blue veins from legs for—ah, heart bypass
surgery? Yes, a heart attack, Elbert confirmed.

Elbert, prudently, wouldn't venture any more into
Philadelphia traffic around the airport, but he did help
by driving me to visit Dad at the closer Camden hospital
several times. Elbert would stop to chat with attendants
stuck in parking lots or patients stranded in waiting rooms,
mustering a Kuan Yin's Contentment Anywhere. Whereas
Dad has always been shy, Elbert was outgoing; Dad,
taciturn, Elbert, talkative; Dad, recently hard of hearing,
Elbert, near deaf for decades. As Dad's voice cracked and
weathered over the years, the brothers had less and less
chance of communicating verbally, but Elbert didn't seem

to mind. From the back door, he'd wave, "Hey, Marvin!" as enthusiastically as ever and wolf down Dad's wet-bottom shoofly pies appreciatively.

No shoofly pies in 1996, nor now, in Honolulu. Dad is flipping through the photographs from the memorial service for Elbert at the stream. "So. George died last week." "Um, Elbert. George died about ten years ago." "That long?" He pauses. "Did George go suddenly?" "Yes, a heart attack." "Last time I saw George, his lips were blue! You knew Something was coming." Actually, Dad's lips have had a faint blue tinge for months now.

While I'm talking to Martha on the phone about the other mourners at the graveside, she tells me not only about blue hands but about Elbert's very first car. The folks at the funeral trotted out the old story of Elbert working at Baumas' farm and maybe strutting a bit over his grand purchase. The Bauma boy liked the new car too and kept trying out its horn, "Ah-oooo-ga." After fifty or so ah-oooo-gas, Elbert took pity on the spooked cows, caught the Bauma boy, and tanned his hide. Now the surviving Phillipses, the old dairy family, and Elbert's long-time truck mechanic at the funeral chortle at the story.

Dad comes worriedly from staring in the bathroom mirror: "My lips are blue." "Yes, they have a slight bluish tinge," I agree cautiously, "but they've been that way for months. It's not a sign of Something right away." He looks relieved.

The Moon in the Water

"That's not the end of the story," Martha says, still reporting the antics at the funeral. The Bauma boy had the last word, so to speak. After his tanning for ah-oooo-ga-ing, he climbed into a tree and pissed exuberantly down onto the new car. The Phillipses, the dairy family, Elbert's long-time truck mechanic—all chortle and dance at the funeral, over the moon.

Calling the Moon

According to surviving reports, famous painter Chou Fang, eighth century, contributed a Water-Moon Kuan Yin for the southeastern wing of a pagoda at Sheng-kuang-su. Chou sketched Kuan Yin's robe in a few bold strokes and then enlivened its folds with wash after wash of colors, tremulously shading into each other. However, some commentators claim that another artist, Liu Ch'eng, must have painted this masterpiece in the pagoda, since the background halo and bamboo, so familiar for Water-Moon Kuan Yins, glowed in single-color blocks, characteristic of Liu, not in Chou's blended tints. Scholars do not know exactly what to call this work: Water-Moon Kuan Yin by Chou Fang? By Liu Ch'eng? In any case, the famous painting by Chou Fang (or Liu Ch'eng, or Chou Fang and Liu Ch'eng together) has now been lost.

My dad's family has always called him Marvin, but when I visited him in the hospital in 1996, after his bypass surgery, I was dismayed to hear the nurses hail him as John. His parents did register him John Marvin, and I suppose it was easier for Billing to follow legality rather than quirk and custom. Yet when it turned out that he was losing so much that summer—his freedom, the use of his left leg, the control of his bowels for two weeks, and the control of his bladder for two months—the additional loss of his name depressed me. "Come on, John, eat your pudding." Who was this John and why should he eat your ol' pudding?

On the other hand, the new incarnation as John started to thrive. In the fall when I went back to Hawai'i, he hired Pat to clean house, a few hours a week, and she always referred to him as John, the heart-patient name. Somehow her drawl opened up vistas between the J and the N, with time to dally past the mysterious H. Pat cooked the ham and cabbage, then sat on the back stoop with Dad, blending her throaty laugh and his appreciative chuckle. Over the next few years, phone conversations told me that if he disappeared briefly into the hospital with more heart pains or suspected pneumonia, it was Pat who visited with Skittles candy, rescued his walker, and smuggled extra trousers when Dad checked himself out against doctor's orders, outwitting the nurse's ruse of "hiding" his pants. Whenever I traveled back to New Jersey, I could see for myself that John's eyes lit up for Pat and her family. As soon as her great-grandson, Daeshawn, poked his head in the back door, the little guy flew, arms reaching, to "Mr. John!"

Once Mr. John has moved from Cinnaminson to Honolulu, his name is Dad again. He's not sure he wants to be here. "Can I go home?" he asks frequently. After a month or so, he grows more content and exclaims periodically, "It's lucky we met up again out here!"

Sometimes he varies this conclusion into "How did we meet up out here?" as if I'm a stranger who has—kindly perhaps, but inexplicably—taken up his cause.

The closing statements for the sale of Dad's house in Cinnaminson finally arrive. The attorneys for the buyer have searched court dockets for Dad's name, to turn up any creditors who might covet the house. A John Phillips, residing in Weehawkin, owes child support to his former wife, residing in Okeechobee. Another John Phillips, aka John Bock, aka Tim Buck, residing in Shamong, owes child support to a woman who lists her name as "Love." A John Phillips (the same, or a different one), residing in Lenape Township, owes Sears, Roebuck, and Company $1,439.62. The shenanigans of these shadow Johns are now stapled to the closing papers, a permanent part of Dad's record.

Somehow, the wayward Johnnies all seem to reside in towns with Native American names. The European settlers, after decimating the original inhabitants through shootings, infections, and shoddy land deals, clutched fast to the names of the conquered: for their mana? Susquehanna and Monongahela still hum over the radio news. Even the name Cinnaminson, Dad's town for fifty years, is conjectured as Senemensing, a Lenni Lenape word meaning "sweet water." In any case, most of the Native Americans, who gave their names and much else besides, are now lost from the area.

What sweet water did the lost ones mean? The polluted Pennsauken Creek in Senemensing? Kapiolani Stream in

The Moon in the Water

Honolulu? Has Kuan Yin spotted the moon in the water? Dad pauses on his meanderings through my apartment and peers at me a long time. Finally he sketches me in: "You're my and Madeline's child!" He doesn't sound sure.

When my friend Mercedes is visiting, I glance into Dad's room to see if he's awake. He's sitting on the edge of the bed. "There he is!" I greet inanely, after his long nap. "There's who? Humpty Dumpty?" he proposes. After asking from the doorway if she can come in, Mercedes flops down cross-legged on the floor and looks up directly into Humpty's face. He instantly trusts her and chats easily, while I fix lunch. Before she leaves in the afternoon, she asks if she can call him "Tatang," father in Ilocano. He looks moved. "So it's okay if I call you Tatang?" Remembering the father's role, among so much that is lost, Dad reassures her, in a suddenly strong voice: "If you need help, call me."

Moon Dung Kuan Yin

An anonymous handout from Comparative Religion 101
has made the rounds on campus: duplicated for classes,
handed on to friends. Its single page sums up twelve
religions in neat squares, all on the theme "Shit happens."
The Zen square ponders its koan, "What is the sound of
shit happening?" and Hinduism sizes up past incarnations,
"This shit has happened before." According to the witty
author, Protestantism holds itself aloof, "Let shit happen
to someone else," while Catholicism harrumphs, "If shit
happens, you deserve it." In the outlook attributed to
Buddhism, "If shit happens, it really isn't shit." Either Kuan
Yin isn't paying attention, or else she *is* delving closely, into
the smelly complexity of things.

When Dad first moved to Honolulu, he relied on deep
blue bottles, white liquid, to keep his bowels working.
He would swallow a spoonful in the evening, and when
it didn't do the trick overnight, gulp down another dose.
This double whammy caught up with him, leaving me to
dunk boxer shorts in a pail and him to sprawl exhausted.
"How about I keep the bottle and pour you some now and
then. . . ."

From my neighboring square, I could maybe tell you a thing or two about shit. Ten years ago, on a visit to Dad in New Jersey, I had an emergency colostomy after a hole opened up in my intestines. I was just strolling along, blue October sky, when I felt a tiny pinprick; five hours later, agony. On the handout, Islam resigns itself to Grand Whim, "If shit happens, it is the will of Allah," while Judaism wonders what "chosen" could have meant, "Why does this shit always happen to us?" In a letter to me in the hospital, a Jewish friend provided the key question about intestines, akin to the one on the page of squares, "Why are they throwing my kishkes around the block?"

The microbiologist who monitored the resulting peritonitis exclaimed excitedly that he had never *seen* the microbes crawling in my gut except in pond samples. Could that really be Kuan Yin's pond? A piece of descending colon emerged as a pursed red fish mouth from a hole poked into my side.

Here in Honolulu, Dad's digestion is not behaving. Hurrying as fast as a walker can leap, he just makes it to the bathroom, then trails little pellets in the hallway. I'm worried because of another memory, six years ago, after his heart bypass surgery, when we had to resort to diapers. No sooner would we change one enormous pad than another would sport a trickle of liquid feces, hardly enough to "get all het up about," he said, but still soiled. One morning, he directed mysteriously, "You'll have to call the airline." "And?" "Leave today." Anybody who didn't know him would think he was firing me, but he was trying to spare his frazzled caregiver. Finally, *he* left, in the middle of the night, by ambulance: bowel obstruction.

The handout from Comparative Religion 101 includes a square for agnosticism, "What is this shit?" and one for atheism, "I don't believe this shit." I wonder how far these tags have circulated: just our campus? Campuses all over the country? Maybe somebody in Normal, Illinois, manuring her fields, had to brake the machine and whip out a notebook to record her sudden twelve insights. The copier before me captured penciled crescent moons, to mark where the squares had hit an answering chord in some anonymous viewer.

The morning after Dad's midnight ride to the hospital, for bowel obstruction, my two former college roommates were scheduled to visit me in New Jersey. Miraculously, Betsy and Shirley came all the way from Massachusetts and Pennsylvania just in time to help with mountains of laundry. I can still see those Kuan Yins laughing, as they wrestled sheets onto the line, the bedclothes and their dresses (identically drop-waist and loose) all billowing in the wind.

Back when my kishkes were throwing themselves around the block, Dad made a perfect nurse. He tracked down an egg-crate mattress because skinniness hurt, he cooked stews, and he put an extension cord on the phone so I could keep it in bed, in case my friends from Hawai'i called. It took three operations, but eventually the doctors

The Moon in the Water

hooked the kishkes together again. After each surgery, Dad would patiently plod with me, as his long-staying houseguest tried walking outdoors again, clutched to his hand in autumn leaves, no leaves, snow.

Here in Honolulu, Dad has weaned himself away from the blue bottles of milky medicine. "I've taken a fancy to these papayas," he says. Papayas and broccoli and green juice (orange juice twirled in the blender with fresh spinach leaves) have helped excretions. A brainstorm: How about his old favorite, pumpkin pudding, for fiber? Along with the eggs and the milk, I throw in cinnamon, ginger, and cloves, wafting the scent of an out-of-season Thanksgiving.

Well, shit happens. The dark yellow piles of pumpkin on our plates look so much like squishy cow pats that I start laughing. "What?" He starts laughing. We're pealing. The cows, the kishkes, fly over the moon.

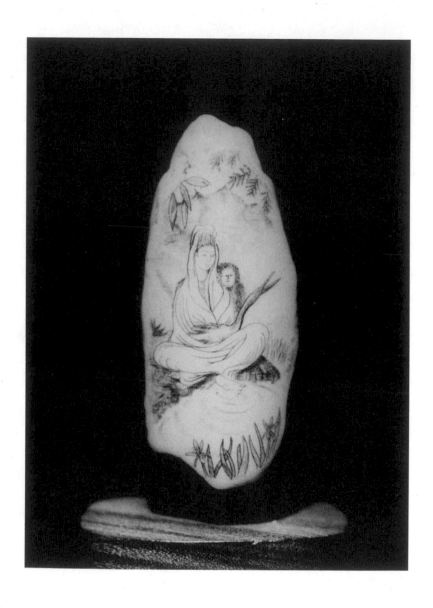

Accidental Moons

Muqi's thirteenth-century "Kuan Yin" hangs in Kyoto,
Japan, between two other scrolls by the same painter:
one of a crane and one of a gibbon with its offspring.
Perhaps the Chinese artist did not originally plan these
three works together, but once a purchaser carried them
all to Japan, and once the temple acquired them and then
displayed them side by side, the accident of their proximity
went on for so long — centuries — that casual visitors and
diligent scholars alike have accepted the three scrolls as
inseparable. What is more, crane, bodhisattva, and gibbon
have interacted over time. They have spun out their own
meaning, which onlookers assume must have been lurking
in Muqi's brush from the first random flick.

   When Dad moves to my Honolulu apartment in June,
I have several months clear to take care of him. As part
of my job at the university, I devote summers to writing;
I can hole up in my study and look in on Dad. As it turns
out, excavating the Medicare card and staking out doctors'
offices do slow my pages, but I can still scribble at odd
moments. When fall comes around, however, we discover
that my class days give Dad too much time alone. He won't
heat up the soup I leave in the refrigerator and he curls up

in a ball. I contact Caregivers' Respite Program to hire a sitter for Monday, Wednesday, and Friday, six hours each.

Muqi's crane, which completely fills the five-foot height of the scroll, looms taller than the white-robed Kuan Yin in the neighboring picture, making a sort of mismatched, feathery beau and bride. Hulda alights on our doorstep from Caregivers' Respite. Although she speaks in a strong Scandinavian accent, she always salutes her way out with "Ciao." Apparently, the last elder whom Hulda helped was a retired military man, and she got in the habit of responding in kind to his idiosyncratic salutes. "Ciao" must have stuck fast from another sojourn entirely.

Hulda spends the day rearranging the pots in the cupboard. I stack them according to what I think of as logic — pots most frequently used, most forward — though I suppose I tossed some of them into their place originally by chance and just repeat the pattern so I don't have to hunt. Hulda follows a pattern different from my own, but just as inflexible: standing crane to the left, seated Kuan Yin in the middle, crouched and impudent gibbons to the right.

Though I grumble about a crane leaving its feathers where it will, I have to admit that Hulda works well with my Dad. She gets him to walk in the lobby, in bursts of energy that I don't seem able to motivate. When I straggle home afternoons, Dad gives an invariable opinion on Hulda: "That's some lady." I take his tone of mingled alarm and praise to mean that he might prefer to hibernate, but, still, he appreciates her dual ability to encourage firmly and

The Moon in the Water

then back off tactfully if he really is too tired to walk. After all, cranes in some systems mean long life.

One Friday Hulda announces, "I won't be here next week. I have to go to the mainland." "You're coming back?" "Of course I'm coming back." After some scrambling, I miraculously get my friend Cheryl to substitute. But on Saturday Hulda calls to say she needs another week. "Shall I start looking for somebody from Caregivers' Respite?" "No, I'm coming back." The following Sunday, at the very last minute, she phones again to say that she won't be back Mondays or Wednesdays, ever, but could do Fridays. I say, "Come this Friday, until I get a permanent replacement." "All right; I'll be there." But she doesn't show up. After six months of total reliability, why did my crane fly the coop in such an awkward takeoff?

Meanwhile, Cheryl pals around with Dad for three weeks. I'm astounded. If this Kuan Yin had said that she couldn't help out, no second possibility followed Cheryl's name on my list. Dad loves her. She brings him plump strawberries. Next she bestows a UNICEF puzzle: Noah's ark, cranes paddling far from the boat. She offers Dad a whole chocolate cake. With his Polaroid, Dad snaps photos of Cheryl. Perhaps he forgets that he took her picture the day before. In any case, we soon have snapshots of Cheryl propped all over the house, like those of a family member through years of development.

Fortunately for Cheryl, our competent Caregivers' Respite Program sends a more regular replacement for

Hulda, named Elise. (Dad calls her Elsie.) She adopts me as her baby gibbon, leaving Lemon Spritzer cookies in the refrigerator with a tag "for K." She chides me for wearing wrinkled shirts and irons them herself, after somehow lugging onto the bus and out to my apartment a heavy ironing board, in morning-glory print. "Elise, put your feet up," I advise futilely. Though in her sixties, she is lithe and energetic and pushes Dad in his wheelchair to their sanctuary under a flowering Chinese orchid tree. They feed sunflower seeds to doves and java-rice birds. She sets Dad apart from her recent charges: "He's so *decent*!"

The commentators on Muqi's "Crane, Kuan Yin, and Gibbons" write that because the flanking pair sidle up to a bodhisattva, they have acquired a Buddhist coloring they might not have had if the Kyoto purchaser had hung each alone, in some prince's hall or lady's chamber. With Kuan Yin nearby, however, the animals seem to chirp or chatter a religious message. One scholar even characterizes the older simian's expression as a "blank, confronting stare . . . that confounds any interpretation," so that the creature's gaze toward the viewer must convey "the unsettling ambiguities of the Ch'an [Zen] encounter." But that scholar reads too much hostility, I think, into the prickliness of the teaching master or the intractableness of a life's experiences. The gambolings a monkeyish fate sends me might be intentionless but not confrontational. And the loops a gibbon traces on my page might be blank to begin with, but they can certainly be filled in.

One day after the recent flux in caregivers, Dad reaches over to shake hands: "I want to thank you for getting me such good babysitters." "Elder-sitters," I mumble, surprised at so formal a thanks. The great and not-so-great sitters line up like the silk panels at a Kuan Yin exhibit, like the members of an accidental family. Even biological family members line up like an accidental artwork. Still, their crotchets and their flights, their frayed feathers and their monkeyshines, go on making meaning. They beget meaning.

Bodhi-Dad

In this picture, Dad sits on a rocky bank. His right foot
crosses his left knee, and his roughened workman's hands
are clasping his ankle. Like Water-Moon Kuan Yin,
he's been confined: cramped in an airplane, plunked on
an island, marooned in a doctor's office, belted into a
wheelchair, locked in illness, backed into old age.

Like Kuan Yin, Dad is also patiently settled on his rock
to hand out boons. It's not always clear in these old prints
who's lapping it up and who's giving, who's doing the lolling
and who, the carrying. Is Kuan Yin helpfully pouring out
the Gatorade? Or is the rock helpfully holding up Kuan
Yin?

Bodhi-Dad gives me several gifts now that he's living
in Honolulu. For one thing, he bestows the great pleasure
of hearing Mom praised. When I ask him how he got to
be so sweet, he shoots back, "Madeline!" If I thank him for
carrying me on school trips, to inspect the ostrich eggs in
the museum, he again credits Madeline: "She knew what
to do. I just kept me mouth shut." "Well, that's a talent in
itself," I tell him. Now that he's old and slowed, he often

marvels at his past good fortune: "I can't believe Madeline picked me out!"

He reflects on his and Mom's values in picking each other. "You hear these kids nowadays talk about 'a nice butt, a nice butt.' Can you make a life with a butt alone?" I duly consider such a life. "No," he answers himself triumphantly, "you have to look for the personality!" Madeline had a Kuan Yin personality, and I don't mean saccharine. She laughed. She sang like a sharma thrush and continued to sing even from hospital beds, before and after her twenty-five-plus operations (hernias, "benign" tumors as big as grapefruit, odd bones). Mom radiated courage, as did her mother before her, yet not quite the same. Whereas Gram had stoicism, Mom had zest. Madeline was clearly the real moon, sailing the sky, while Dad and I, lesser puddles, learned to emit our little light as amazed reflections of her.

If Dad caught his cue for Kuan-Yin parenting from Mom, he carried on the part with little prompting. When I was eleven, a neighbor girl, sixteen, moved in with us because she wasn't getting along with her family. Maureen took a new interest in school, then turned out to be skipping class to see her boyfriend instead, and, oops, got pregnant. When Mom told Dad about this latest snag in raising daughters, his very first reaction — not second thoughts or a later smoothing over — was to say hopefully,

"It'll be nice having a kid around the house again." By contrast, her real father hit her. In a state of permanent hysteria, Maureen's parents sent her to a home for unwed mothers, made her quit school to support the child, and let the TV babysit for years. If only the family had realized, they could have had Bodhi-Dad use daylight hours freed by the night shift on the railroad to keep the kid company.

Dad did keep company with Florence, his mother-in-law. She had moved in with my parents in her eighties and, after Madeline died, continued to live with Marvin for seven more years. They made a good team. Dad cooked—his everything-but-the-kitchen-sink stews in a pink glass pot—and Gram did the dishes. She kept herself occupied cutting out squares for patchwork quilts and stitching them together on her old treadle machine, preserving remnants from dresses she'd made for Mom and me in the old days. Because Gram couldn't see very well, ordinary delays in the task, like the needle coming unthreaded, stretched into long, silent struggles. She preferred to stab the air alone rather than "bother" Dad for help. He took to strolling past her room now and then, sauntering in to rethread the needle as if he just *happened* to be passing.

Now in Hawai'i, Dad *happens* to wander off to his bedroom when the three members of my writing group arrive, so as not to inhibit our reading. The group members listen to "No Moon," wonder what "no moon" means, and suggest that my only Irish ancestors, who bequeathed my family the word "shillelagh," may have been denizens of 1950s' television programs, Arthur Godfrey and Carmelle Quinn. I do vaguely recall those names; what a comedown for a genealogy. "How kind of your Dad to make himself scarce while the writing group meets," someone says. Make himself scarce—the common phrase brings tears to my eyes. No doubt we are all, along with Kuan Yin's moon, getting full, getting scarce, getting gone.

Roundabout Moon

Kanō Kōi's "White-Robed Kannon," from sixteenth-century Japan, clearly derives from the water-moon type. Like some nesting bird, this Kuan Yin (in her Japanese name) fluffs her robes over a stony outcropping, a mere four-foot drop to the water. If she lost her balance, a fall would seem safe enough, by distance — though she'd better not land on that large rock with eddies around it. Next to her, rainwater has collected in an accidental basin of stone. From time to time she glances into the basin, or into the bay, waiting to catch the reflections of moon.

In Honolulu, I like hearing Dad say aloud the appreciation for Mom that had (over the years) always been tacit. It's not that I ever doubted his affection for her or for me either. But since he always expressed himself indirectly before, the difference is like seeing the colors arch so easily through the rain in Hawai'i, whereas rainbows had just been theoretic possibilities back in New Jersey. On the other hand, outright rainbows run the risk of co-option, to greeting card cliché. So now I'm leaning toward putting in a good word for Dad's old indirection too.

Like a Kuan Yin painting, Dad communicated silently. He knew without my saying that his tiny child dreaded escalators, so he would take my hand without comment. If his grad school daughter insisted on spending the entire Christmas vacation holed up in the unheated attic (since Gram had my old room), Dad required no explanation. Studying might not appeal to him, but he respectfully guarded its appeal to me. I'd hear a tap at the door of my retreat, then a hand would appear in the small space between doorjamb and table, deposit a plate with cut-up apple pieces next to the books on the bench, and withdraw without a word.

In "White-Robed Kannon," sixteenth-century Kanō has dashed off her robe in quick strokes of pale ink. The fluid waves below echo the folds of the robe, harmonizing woman and world. The artist has left her high headdress austerely blank; usually it emblazons Amida Buddha, but Kanō prefers to acknowledge the unpicturable. Fully one half of the hanging scroll rises empty around her.

Communicating by deed and demeanor, Dad watched me first move away from home without a fuss. This was the summer before my senior year in high school. I'd been spending a week with Mom and Gram at Ephrata, Pennsylvania, where we went for a week every summer for meditation and classes. The cashier in the dining room had quit, and when Dad drove up to take us back to New Jersey, I bounded out to the car: "Hey, Dad, they want me to stay on and work!" "Okay." Nothing about "This will be your first time on your own." Nothing like "Do you think you can do it?" Instead, he drove me into downtown Ephrata to purchase an alarm clock and a back brush, carted my plaid suitcase up to the fourth floor where the help roomed, and disappeared down the road with Mom and Gram. As I interpreted all their versions of tactful restraint, Mom knew I'd be fine and shared my excitement, Gram prudently refrained from interfering, and Dad worried more (or so I surmised from his face) but still did not dump extra cautions.

Even though Kanō gives more than half his paper scroll to empty space, he does write his signature. The vertical characters dangle in a clump, like the wisteria blossoms Dad planted over his porch back in Cinnaminson. And the eddies overlap a red, rectangular seal. The two sets of characters, black and red, comprise the only words reflected on his pale water swirls.

At twenty-three or so, I sent Dad a letter (I admit it; sometimes I choose the rainbow right out), trying to list the good things I'd learned from him. I recorded, for example, my admiration at his spontaneous response to Maureen's unplanned pregnancy, "It'll be nice having a kid around the house." While he didn't directly acknowledge my letter, Mom reported that he had taken it to the copier at the firehouse and duplicated it—twice. He gave one copy to Mom. "Who's the other one for?" Oh, he'd keep the second one too, he said, to supplement the original, because "it might wear out." Kuan Yin duplicates her moon, from basin to bay, to open ocean.

The Moon in the Water

Kuan Yin's Taxable Domain

Kuan Yin presides on a ledge jutting over an inlet. Three stalks of bamboo shoot up behind her, flecking her with skimpy shade. A willow branch sticks out of a cruet on a dirt mound. Across the waves, a girl with arms outstretched stands on an island; on another island, a boy holds up an incense burner. In this dashed-off sketch, a haphazard bird flies past Kuan Yin and the moon.

When Dad moves in with me, I take over the task of filing his income tax forms. The first year, I do my taxes in February, but after slaving over my own calculations, I can't bear to look at his papers right away. At the last minute I scribble in his numbers, expecting no trouble from his modest income, a railroad pension. "Fill in line 12a from Form RRB-1099-R." Wait; we have no Form 1099-R. Recalling the long effort to extract Dad's Medicare card with red stripe from the august Railroad Retirement Board, I give up all hope of obtaining Form 1099-R before the tax deadline. I check a square that says, "Let the IRS figure your tax for you." As I briefly report my efforts to Dad, he empties his box of Crispy Wheats ("Any more of them flats?") and nonchalantly predicts that this "letting" the IRS do anything will cost us "a pretty penny."

Kuan Yin's willow bears only three leaves. And what

is that branch doing in a vessel with spout? She needs a vase, not a kettle. Or maybe she's planning to steep tea in her kettle. But what kind of balm is she brewing with three measly leaves? Please, Kuan Yin; let's get more practical.

I write the Railroad Retirement Board and politely request that it put us down to receive a Form 1099-R next year. The board replies, most contrite, that it did send us a form this year but, alas, omitted our apartment number. The clerk assures me that he or she has now entered the whole address, the complete address, the correct address into the computer.

As sure as the waning of the moon, the new tax year rolls around. I am delighted to have received for Dad both Form RRB-1099-R and Form SSA-1099, from the Social Security Administration. Comfortably shaded by these fluttering pages, I sit down to fill out Dad's Tax Form 1040A. However, at the obvious line for his information, 12a, Pensions and Annuities, I am once again stumped. It turns out that railroad pensions differ from almost every other pension in the U.S. of A., in that the railroad check *folds in* Social Security benefits. I consult the instruction booklet: "See Pub. 575 to find out how to report your benefits." Kuan Yin has one vessel with spout, one willow branch, and four bamboo stalks. She does not have Pub. 575, though she may be ready for a swig or two.

I try looking for Pub. 575 on the Internet the next day at school. Sure enough, I can click my way forward. Since I don't have much time before class, I ask my miraculous

The Moon in the Water

computer to print pages seven through eleven of Pub. 575, relevant to railroad workers. Unfortunately, my miraculous computer misreads the page numbers and gives me five identical copies of one irrelevant worksheet, all blank lines.

It's hard to tell if Kuan Yin's attendants across the waves are bringing her gifts or begging them from her. The boy with arms raised could be offering "your tax dollars at work," the usual sign planted next to the heaps of gravel impeding my progress down the walkway. After all, this boy seems to be holding a kind of incense burner, the contents going up in smoke. By contrast, the other figure, with arms out, has no offering. She seems to be asking Kuan Yin's contribution, a large contribution: Solve my life for me. Or, more likely, she's yelling: Pay for my war.

Okay, better not make my war protest through Dad's tax form: "Eighty-Year-Old Arrested for Refusal to Pay War Tax, Jailed at Isolated Inlet." The news item will read, "Speaking from Guantanamo by cell phone, which he has never used before and so must rely on the non-POW, noncitizen, non-noncitizen, eighteen-year-old hooded Taliban soldier beside him to operate, the octogenarian WWII veteran rasps out that all wars are stupid, but this thing about invading Iraq just about takes the cake, and darned if he's going to fork over any of his RRB or SSA benefits for it."

Uncowed, Kuan Yin has been fermenting her three measly willow leaves with the bamboo leaves to make a nice soothing drink. The next day at school, when I have more time, I read Pub. 575 online, rather than try to print it out. The screen tells me that one of the squares on Form RRB-1099-R includes an SSEB, the Social Security Equivalent Benefit lodged *inside* a railroad pension. Another square records a NSSEB, a non–Social Security Equivalent Benefit, which "may be partly taxable." But nothing on this screen tells me how to judge which parts of Dad's SSEB or NSSEB are and are not taxable.

By now Kuan Yin is pretty high on her fermented concoction, something like the dandelion wine Gram used to make after getting Dad to help her pick yellow dandelion blossoms into a pillow case. Kuan Yin says casually, "Look, we still have this moon. Use the light from that." Okay, here's a pertinent piece of information in the instruction booklet back home. Add the number from Box 5 of RRB-1099-R and the number from Box 5 of SSA-1099, divide the sum by two, and compare the number to $25,000. Is your number bigger or smaller? Ah, an answer of which I am capable. My number is smaller. Then "none of your Social Security benefits are taxable." Hooray!

Of course, we still have to figure which part of the pension *per se* is taxable.

Did I tell you Kuan Yin's moon bird is flying upside down?

I wing my way back to the screen at school. It says to add the box on RRB-1099-R for Vested Dual Benefit and the box for Contributory Amount Paid and put *that* sum on line 12a, Pensions and Annuities. I add in some "aughts"

The Moon in the Water

(as Dad calls them) to compute his AGI (adjusted gross income). "Subtract Standard Deduction (see left margin) from AGI." The answer is—um—less than zero. Hooray! Dad needs to toss no tax across the waves.

So, that $500 we tossed last year when we let the IRS figure for us *did* amount to a "pretty penny," quite a potent shower of them.

What's this? Next on the heap: Form N-11, Dad's Hawai'i State Tax Form. The difference here is that if you are past sixty-five, you can claim yourself as your responsibility twice, which sure enough sounds like something you forgot you already did once. Or, as Dad would put it, "Once't or twice—give 'er a go."

Slim Pickings/Fat Moon

Kuan Yin is hunched on a dirt mound on her tiny island. The cramped land is just big enough to support four spindly bamboo stalks, chopped off and sharp pointed. Barefooted, she has wedged her jar beside her: no willow, no water. She has a circle round her head and a bigger one — the moon — round her whole body. One sutra says that the curve round her head is a "halo," containing "five-hundred Bodhisattvas and countless devas [spirits]," while the ring circling her body is a "nimbus," holding "the five species of sentient beings." Nevertheless, a commentator on this sutra admits that "for all practical purposes," artists may continue to paint Kuan Yin with blank halo and nimbus: a couple of pen strokes, modest and unpopulated.

Dad and I are walking around the house warily, on the verge of rejoicing but still suspicious. He is free of pain now, but last evening, from five until midnight, some sharp point kept jabbing into a spot on his lower back. The pain would ease up, then dart back, with a strong enough prod to make him cry out. Were his kidneys quitting? No, this morning they're still working. Though he feels okay now, we set up an appointment with the doctor.

I call a cab and fetch Dad his shoehorn. Gazing at

the irregularly pounded iron, in no hurry for his shoes, he recounts that great-granddaddy H. handmade this shoehorn. For some reason, I've never heard this origin for the familiar object. I did know the lore that great-granddaddy worked as a carpenter in the Pennsylvania coal mines, building props to shore up the earth. I remember the man, smoking a meerschaum pipe. I remember his funeral—open casket, sharp nose—when I was four. In his lifetime, he coerced his son, my grandpa, to quit school in the eighth grade to work on the farm. Kunkel always bitterly resented this theft of his education. Kunkel courted my future Gram in a horse-drawn buggy, from Wilkes Barre, Pennsylvania (pronounced Wilkes Bury, as in "buried in the mines"). The newspaper, just this morning, in fact, is carrying a story of nine miners trapped in a Pennsylvania mine. The horse and buggy, the casket, the mines (then and now), all come trailing out of the bluish blotches on the iron shoehorn. Kuan Yin is contemplating her toes on a tiny island, no shoes in sight.

I'm sure our cab has come and gone. Eventually, Dad deigns to ease on his sneakers. We make our cab. At the doctor's, Dad can't exactly remember the pain (fortunately, I guess), so I describe its arabesques. The doctor says it sounds like Dad passed a small kidney stone. To confirm her diagnosis and check for any infection, she gives us a jar to collect his first urine of the next day and carry it, in a plastic pouch, to a lab in our neighborhood.

Back home with this good news ("good" in the sense

that the hard stone has moved to past tense), we're a lot closer to rejoicing. I offer to help with his bathing, but he says, "I'd just as leave take a nap." Out of the blue, I suddenly recognize in his usual expression "just as leave" the medieval phrase "just as lief." My old dad has survived from the fourteenth century! His archaic speech conjures up a caparisoned horse and a jeweled sword, or rather (the social class in which I'd likely run into us), a serf grasping his pitchfork to delve in the earth or swinging his curved blade to reap. Come to think of it, Dad did still have a rusty sickle in the cellar when we scoured out his belongings before he moved here.

At this point, Kuan Yin is amusing herself by doing a handstand on the back of the dolled-up medieval horse. (Okay, so she's pretending she's a Minoan handstander on the backs of bulls.) When she falls off that creature (one of a subset of the "five species of sentient beings"), she makes friends with the other horse on the scene, the one patiently hitched to a tree while my grandparents do a little spooning. Politely, she offers the horse an apple; delicately, the horse gathers it in with its velvety lips. At the center of the circling halo, nimbus, and lake (her three-ring circus), Kuan Yin tries a few somersaults in place.

When I hear Dad getting up at six the next morning, I leap out of bed to offer our clean jar. We cap our specimen triumphantly. When the lab opens at eight-thirty, I stroll over, but the technician eyes our sample skeptically: "Has it been out of the refrigerator for more than half an hour?"

"Uh, yeah." "No good." Kuan Yin, nobody told me to *refrigerate* your jar! The technician tucks a new empty jar plus sheathed towelette in the zipper pocket and the doctor's request in the back pocket of the plastic pouch, stamped "Globalpak." Small world.

I'm poised all day to hand Dad the fresh jar, with a plan to carry the precious drops, bottled, in a bag of ice cubes. "Think we'll get our sample?" "Can't never tell." Output is slight on this island. Would you believe he doesn't urinate again until 6 p.m.? The lab, of course, closes at 5:30.

Our whole life is focused on one pot of piss, and now we don't even have that. I'm hoping that collecting a specimen is just not important any more. The pains are past, though still lodged in at least one of our memories. During that evening of fierce jabs, whenever he'd yell out, I'd dash into his room. Finally he said, "Are *you* holding up okay?" Now, there's one of your five hundred Bodhisattvas, right there, in the curve of the moon.

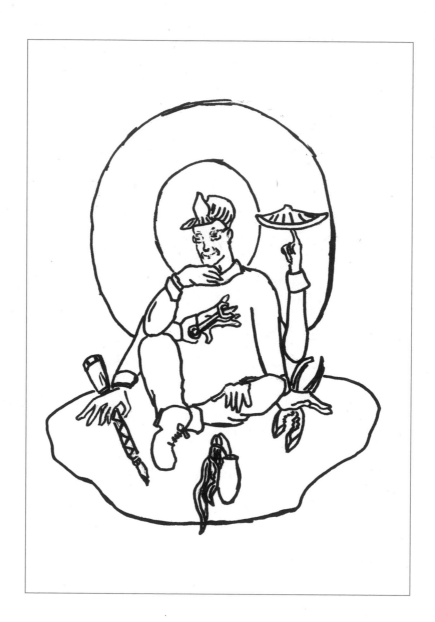

Moon Rings

The "Wheel-Turning Kannon" in this fifteenth-century Japanese hanging scroll definitely follows the water-moon type. A male figure is lounging on a light-filled lotus, with right knee drawn up close to the body and left leg bent flat. A halo frames the head, while the larger, concentric moon curves around the whole body. Dressed in loose pants, he looks relaxed and homey, except for an extravagant six arms, borrowed from some Hindu god preceding Buddhism. "Wheel" in the title must mean the dharma wheel of the law, but it looks in the picture like a top (spinning on a pinky), perpendicular to the ring round his head. The artist has anchored the whole composition in browns and dark greens, except for touches of glowing gold here and there and the almost miraculously lustrous pink of the lotus.

Kuan Yin will need all six arms to keep straight the story of a John, a John Marvin, and a Jonette. About two years before Dad (the John Marvin) moved to Honolulu, he scrawled from New Jersey the minor news that a theater troupe had bought my old kindergarten building. I wrote back that, yes, I recalled that place and year very well. There I learned that my odd bones might pose a few problems ("buttons coat" on my first report card earned a big "U" for Unsatisfactory), but at the same time I grasped that those bones could give gifts. In kindergarten, I received the still-vivid boon—vivid enough to include in the letter to Dad—of seeing classmate John Pelham delicately fastening the wooden barrel buttons on my gray woolen coat as I gazed down at his long, dark, slender, amazing, five-year-old fingers.

At the time of our exchange of letters about kindergarten, Dad was in the thick of a friendship with a twelve-year-old from the neighborhood, Jonette Parry. She had veered her bicycle into his driveway and screeched to a halt in front of his garage one day and struck up a conversation. Over the months, Dad let her take the shortcut through his yard to the back lot of fireflies, lent her his pliers, listened to her after-school chatter, and refrained from reproaching her for smoking: "No sense in hollerin'." At home on a tidy lotus pad, he spun the spokes of a bicycle wheel with one hand, as another hand tightened up a screw.

For some reason, Dad read my letter about John Pelham's long fingers to his housekeeper, Pat. It turned out that Pat stored a whole history of John Pelham, extending way past my kindergarten memory. Dad duly repeated her words in his next letter, so that one of Kuan Yin's arms crossed quietly to connect John Pelham with Jonette—his daughter. Though her different last name had failed to clue us, there it was, that unlikelihood. Another of Kuan Yin's arms gently lifted John Pelham after a fall from a roof, his body dead at scarcely forty, when Jonette was two. John Marvin then shared the letter about John's miraculous coat-buttoning hands with Jonette herself, who seemed tickled by this glimpse of a dad younger than she.

I met Jonette myself on a few visits to New Jersey. She had the most lustrous skin I have ever seen: a dark mahogany, like Pelham's, with an uncanny glow. She was clearly good to my dad. She would slither into the crawl space to fetch an old album, trundle out the trash can on a lawnmower he had fitted with crescent-shaped struts, and add an enthusiastic "Hey, Marvin!" to his day. But the last time I saw her, they'd had a falling out. Somebody told Dad that Jonette got in trouble with the police for pushing down an old woman and snatching her purse. I argued with him that either the rumor was untrue (as I thought), or she'd messed up (as he thought) but wouldn't continue on that route (I said) if she kept buddies like him. They hadn't visited in quite a while. Still, when she heard by the grapevine that he was moving to Hawai'i, she biked over to say goodbye. "Dad, it's Jonette! Do you want to come out to the living room?" "No. I ain't home." I sat on the back stoop and lied to Jonette: He's asleep. Did he feel that she had pushed down all old people, including him? Or did he clutch fast such rumors because, otherwise, moving away from this surrogate daughter would be loss too great to bear?

Staring now at the "Wheel-Turning Kannon," I can see a lot of wear and tear in the silk. Yet as I inspect the small halo around the head, it dawns on me that the larger "moon" is really a halo too, the radiance projected from the teacher. The identity of moon and self must have been there all along, in all of the pictures, in all of our poses, as we go on landing and losing Kuan Yin's role in our small-town theater. We all give out our little light, not just once, but in repeated rings, like a pulse, like the ripples in a pool. That Water-Moon Kuan Yin—she has the moon, she has the water, right inside.

The Moon in the Water

Kuan Yin Foot Dangler

Kuan Yin is dangling her foot from an overhanging bank. Her willow sprig in its cup has dried to a brittle brown. Still, her bamboo stalks are thriving, swaying and creaking at a new spindly height. The moon, three-quarters through its cycle, leans with horns pointing right. At 5 a.m., the moon stoops, bleary eyed, but still emits a glow, a firefly surprise. And at the edge of its ring, what an amazing, exuberant, burnished bronze!

"How long am I going to be able to bum off of you?" Dad asks. "Not bumming," I protest. "Look, you peel the potatoes, right?" He is pleased whenever I set the cutting board at his place. He disdains the scraper and guides a knife with his big hands, piling up long strips of brown or rose potato peel. As a kid I liked to watch him pare an apple, transforming the skin into one long, patient spiral, dangling down.

"Do you have access to my money?" Dad wants to know. "Yes, from the joint account. You were smart to set that up," I congratulate him. Back when he was still in New Jersey, a young woman hired after his defibrillator operation discovered she could tell him she "needed help," and he'd write her a check—many checks. He didn't remember he'd already written a "gift" check to Letitia the day before. In this manner, she defrauded him of $700. Though the police looked for Letitia, the scumbag had already scrammed.

"Hey, Kathy, how much would you want for room and board?" "Three hugs a month," I demand, moving closer for an installment. He readily pays a hug but looks unconvinced. Kuan Yin's bamboo bums its CO_2 off Kuan Yin. Kuan Yin bums her oxygen off bamboo.

"Do you have access to my money?" Dad asks. "Yes, the joint account." An outsider might think he took me for Letitia, depleting his funds. But I know the next question: "Am I paying my fair share?" I reassure him: "You pay for your medicines. You pay for your food. You pay your medical premium." He looks doubtful: "Is that enough rent?" "You don't have any rent, because I'd be paying that anyway, whether you were here or not." "Oh." The chloroplasts in Kuan Yin's bamboo leaves, which use her CO_2, live inside the bamboo cells independently. These chloroplasts have their own DNA, which turns out to resemble the DNA of bacteria more than the DNA of a plant. At some point in the distant past, the chloroplasts moved into plant cells, in symbiosis.

"Hey, Kathy, how much would you want for room and board?" "Don't worry. You pay your way. It's not everybody who has a private secretary," I boast, handing Dad a small stack of printer paper. He looks pleased, my secretary, and starts carefully tearing the perforated edges. I bought this brand for my old printer. Then the computer to which the printer was tethered conked out. The new computer wouldn't speak to my old printer, in tip-top shape though it was. I had to get a new printer, one that feeds on edgeless paper only. When Dad saw me tearing on the dotted line, he pounced on a new job "for my keep."

"Do you have access to my money?" Dad asks. "Yes, you

pay your way. Plus I need three hugs a month." Dad laughs as he reaches out: "Did I ask you that before?" The mitochondria in human cells, which allow oxygen to be used, live inside Kuan Yin's cells independently. Like chloroplasts, mitochondria have their own DNA, which resembles the DNA of bacteria more than the DNA of animals. At some point in the ancient days, the mitochondria moved into animal cells: strangers living together. Kuan Yin's body cells bum their oxygen-fueled energy off the stranger mitochondria.

"Do you have access to my money?" Dad asks. He is sitting on the edge of his bed, one sock dangling. When he wakes up in the morning, all stiffness and creaking bones, he can pull on one sock but not the other, so I distract him from money by asking if I can help. He or Mom used to put my socks on for me because I don't fold up; as a child, whenever I requested, "Would you put my socks on?" he'd say, "I don't think they'll fit." No matter how many times I asked, he'd still think the joke was funny. Now I think the joke was profound. Whose feet? Who's me?

"Hey, Kathy? If I decide to move in with you," he proposes (after two years here), "is that all right with you?" "That's a good idea," I agree and then add, "Will thinks that's a good idea too. Will says, 'Before Marv came, I had to live in a tiny drawer! That was *boring*!'" Dad laughs. He's always amazed that the doll still speaks, after all these years. Will bums his freedom from Marv.

Kuan Yin on her tiny embankment is eating a shave ice, flavored mochi black bean. Her tides bum their turns off the moon. The moon bums its glow off the sun. The sun . . .

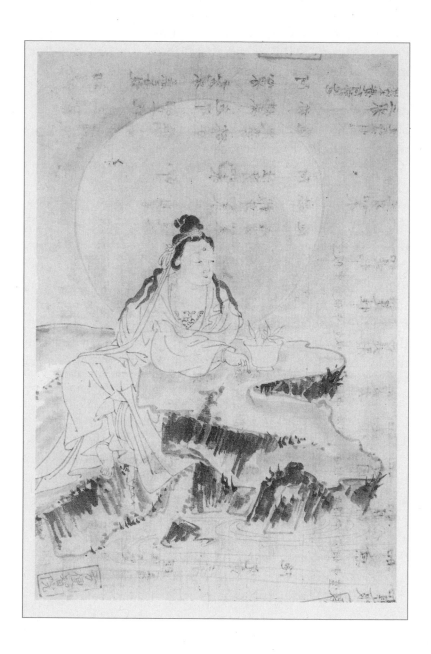

ER Moon

Convenient ledges of rock let this nonchalant Kuan Yin
prop her feet and lean an elbow. The artist has inked her
in on the back of a Buddhist sutra, and its characters show
through dimly, in reverse, on her water, sky, rock, and full
moon; Will might say those letters don't know whether
they're coming or going! Next to her willow sprigs, Kuan
Yin is leaning a finger on the rock; I can't tell if she is
drumming it impatiently, or just keeping her place in the
poem, while she checks for reflections of the moon — and
the verse — in the water.

Dad's caregiver (a new girl) calls school to say he fell
down in his bedroom and cut his head. Because she insists
the cut has stopped bleeding, I wait until after my class to
go home. Only after the caregiver leaves do I notice that
Dad is not putting his weight on his right leg when he
moves to his wheelchair, so at 7 p.m. I call a cab to take us
to the emergency room.

At the hospital the nurse spots Dad's defibrillator and
orders an EKG. I tell her he's not complaining of his heart
and always has unusually low blood pressure, but she hooks
him up anyway. After that test we wait half an hour for the
doctor. Unfortunately, all the movement from wheelchair

to cab (in a rain shower) and from cab to wheelchair (under sprinkles) and from wheelchair to gurney has opened up the cut on his forehead, so it distracts the doctor from my questions about the right leg. While he sews six stitches over Dad's eye, I ask Dad if he remembers taking me to the ER as a kid to get stitches over my eye: "Not hardly." He was calm then and he's calm now, and I don't remind him that I made a lot more noise through my stitching.

"He's not putting his weight on his right leg," I say again to the doctor. While he probes the leg, Dad keeps craning his neck to see what's going on. "Is your neck sore?" the doctor asks. "Kind of"—from all that peering, I suspect. Nevertheless, the doctor orders a CT scan for the neck. "No, no," I protest, "he needs an X-ray of his right leg." The white-coated, unshaven doctor looks doubtful: "Hip maybe. Old people are often breaking hips."

Two aides wheel Dad to the CT room. We wait there forty-five minutes while I drum my fingers impatiently and Dad looks nonchalant. Then we wait for the test to run. Then we wait outside the X-ray room another twenty minutes. When the technicians finally get to him, they shoo me out.

Finally we're finished at the hospital. After I call a cab from the front desk, we station ourselves outside. Half an hour later the cab pulls up. "I can't fit a wheelchair in my trunk!" the cabbie fusses. (I did tell the dispatcher we needed a trunk big enough to accommodate a wheelchair.) As this cabbie, leaving in a huff, does not specify if he'll

The Moon in the Water

signal a new dispatch, I wheel the chair back inside and call a cab again. We return to our curb. Finally the security guard, who's been sauntering in and out of sight, says there's a cab waiting on the other side of the building: Could that be ours? (I did tell the dispatcher 'Ewa side.) I push the wheelchair through the building to Diamond Head side. This cab is still there, and all our selves and our appendages fit into it.

When a hospital official calls the next day to report that the CT scan was fine (I knew that), I learn that allowing myself to be expelled from Dad's little bubble at X-ray was a big mistake. The official adds, "X-ray of left hip also fine." "What? Left hip? But I told every new nurse, doctor, aide who came into the room that it was his right leg!" "I'm sure you did." Pause. "Hold on." The official comes back in about ten minutes: "The X-ray technician says that the order was for left side, but the patient did complain of right, so they did both." I'm not sure whether to believe him. Do these guys know whether they're coming or going? But since Dad's been moving his right leg a little better today, I don't pursue the matter.

The bill comes from the hospital. The ER visit cost $2,195.45. (Insurance—that is, funds from Dad's and everyone's premiums—covers 80 percent.) Within the grand total, the unnecessary CT scan cost $805. The EKG cost $169. First lesson: talk back to doctors and nurses. Do not blend into the background and do make noise, though you think that's your childhood self. It's not. The radiology department charged $400 to X-ray the wrong leg and *possibly* the correct one in addition, though *possibly* not, and *possibly* not the applicable portion of that leg. Next lesson: talk back to radiologists. Do not blend into the background and do not leave Dad alone with them when they try to shoo you out of the room. Categorically *refuse* some treatments (even if it means signing papers in triplicate promising not to sue later) and *insist* on attention to whatever is actually hurting.

Anything else besides rueful lessons to come out of this visit? Dad did give up the walker. Anything positive? Well, he did get six stitches for a cut that was oozing at the moment (though it may not have opened up again if we'd stayed home). And when it came time to take out the stitches, I did not have to deal with the trekking and the tracking of competencies, because my neighbor Nora (the nurse) offered to remove the stitches. She came up from her apartment , got out her scissors, sterilized them, swabbed the skin with alcohol, and snipped out the threads as Dad sat on the edge of his bed. I have to admit that not having to travel to the lair of the experts is one of the gifts I have received most gratefully over the years.

Oh, and the day of the accident, I did get a grand sight. When we finally slouched home from the hospital at 11:30 p.m., I stared out the window for a while. Eventually I registered that the full moon, out from behind a cloud, was reflecting on the puddles in the tennis court, painting them white. Hey, the Moon in the Water!

The Moon in the Water

Kuan Yin Shopper

Sitting on her tiny island, Kuan Yin has four bamboo stalks behind her, sometimes three. Inspect dozens of scrolls; you'll find four stalks, four stalks, four stalks, three. This island is kind of boring, Kuan. What, you don't think so?

After Dad loses control of his excretions in July 2004, shopping for supplies changes the whole meaning of "necessities." Basically, we need Longs-brand underwear, sixteen-count, large. I can take the #6 bus from school, get off after the Japanese Cultural Center, and walk to Longs Mō'ili'ili. I can't purchase too many supplies at once, though. With just two packages, I hardly fit on the bus. Even at seventy-eight pounds, I'm now a "wide load," as Dad would say. And when the bus is crowded, forget it.

Sometimes generous friends offer to pick up supplies for me. But it's better to go with them, because giving instructions is more esoteric than preaching the sutras on a mountaintop. For example, get "underwear," not "briefs." Get sixteen-count, first choice, eighteen-count, second choice. No, don't get eighteen-count *at all* if it says "super-absorbent." The sixteen-count is already thicker and more absorbent, for nighttime, whereas eighteen-count is less absorbent, for daytime. But some eighteen-count, with a yellow stripe, pretend to be "super-absorbent" too, even in the daytime. They're not "super." Why? Because they gap open at the legs. Why does that matter? Because the shishi runs out. What, you no know not'ing?

Get Longs-brand underwear, not Depends. No, not dependable. They gap at the legs too. We know what that means.

Get some underpads. Get Longs-brand, in a dark red package. Sulky red. Get "extra large," not "super large"! "Super large" is larger than "extra large," but "super large" is more square. "Extra large" is more rectangular. A rectangle reaches across the bed better than a square does.

Also, you could get a package of blue, non-Longs-brand underpads, "regular size." Regular is not big enough to be a real underpad, but it's a cheaper way to put a little extra protection under his back, in case the shishi soaks upward on his shirt.

Who'll take me for supplies? A couple of times, Chong. Occasionally, Val. A number of times, Judith. Innumerable times, Suzanne. During the two months of summer when she's here, Perle. My colleague Ruth gives us the maxim for all this: "It takes a village to care for an elder."

Where shall we go? We used to like Longs Mānoa because the green Mānoa hills soothe us all. But Longs Mānoa stopped carrying Longs-brand adult "incontinence supplies." (Word "diaper" not in use.) So we go to Longs Moili'ili. What? All out of sixteen-count! Is someone hoarding? Is the barge late? Ask the clerk. No, nothing in the back. Well, at least get these sulky red packages of Longs-brand underpads, extra large.

What else sits on Kuan Yin's island? A jar. Jar with willow. Jar without willow. Jar on ledge. Jar in hand. If you want a jar to drink out of, it's sure to be filled with greenish water and willow stems. No, thanks.

Want to try Longs Kaimuki? Off we go. Ah, Longs Kaimuki has sixteen-count. Wait, what's this? Longs-brand sixteen-count "reclosable." "Reclosable" means two sides to wrap up and a Velcro patch to close them; they're not the pull-up kind. Simmy (Dad's most recent and truly wonderful helper) can use the reclosable ones okay when I'm at school, but I'm not good at getting them on right. Okay, get *one* reclosable.

After one whole year of buying a forest's worth of expensive diapers, a Longs clerk asks me, "Do you want to apply for a Longs discount card for seniors?" Silent gnashing of teeth, audible "Yes, thank you." Six more weeks for the card.

Kuan Yin is checking the inventory on her island. Three bamboo stalks, one jar, no willow, and — yes! — one cellophane bag of Pui Mui from Longs Moili'ili! What, you no know Pui Mui? Crack seed. Okay, it's Chinese preserved plum. Mmmm!

But don't get the package in a net bag, with the Pui Mui strung together as a lei. Too dry. Get da kine, you know, plum with licorice, *triple*-wrapped: first in clear paper, then in white paper, then in purple, with twisted ends, *then* all the individually wrapped Pui Mui in a cellophane package. Well, yes, there is a pit in each one; just be careful not to chomp down on it. But do gnaw every last scrap from the pit! And for toothless Dad: one pint Häagen-Dazs vanilla.

Car-Key Kuan

A hanging scroll from Korea shows one of the few Water-Moon Kuan Yins I have seen in person. Or maybe I should say, more accurately, "This hanging scroll from Korea *doesn't* show a Water-Moon Kuan Yin I have *almost* seen in person." What an irony. No intervening photographic equipment to blur her jar, no mediating printing process to distort her topknot, and the glimpse is more remote than ever. The exhibit came all the way from Korea to Honolulu and the silk is so sooty I can just about detect a seated Kuan Yin with one ankle resting on the other knee and a Buddhist rosary hanging from his hand. (Korean Kuan Yin, called Kwanseum, is male, but who can pick out such fine distinctions as *he* or *she,* under charcoal?) Or maybe I'm only taking an imaginative leap from the confident words on the wall plaque, and the scroll really pictures an out-of-work chauffeur, ankle crossed on other knee, car keys dangling from an idle hand.

Car-key days with my dad are the worst. Usually he naps on and off, but on car-key days he doesn't sleep a wink. Usually he's taciturn, smiling. On car-key days he talks nonstop and frowns. Usually he is mild-mannered, accommodating, shaking my hand in congratulation because I brought him some ice cream: "You caught my thought!" But on car-key days he is revved up, anxious, raring to go — raring to go some place he should have been yesterday.

You can always tell a car-key day because it starts out, "Where are my car keys?" "Dad, you gave away your van." "Not the van. My black car." That black car rolled sixty years ago, with a running board. (I've seen the one photo of it, next to a goat in the countryside, with great-uncle Ed and grandpa Alonzo throwing back their heads and laughing at some joke I'm not getting.) "Did you take my car keys?" Dad demands; "George is waitin' on me!" George is his oldest brother, dead for more than a decade now. It's clearly a young George waiting, and none too patiently either.

At first I try to set Dad straight. "George died," or "Pat has the van." These facts stick about as well as the mud the wheels fling up, gone by the next spin. Then I get smart. Actually, I would never have gotten smart on my own, if the elderly woman who sits in her folding chair facing busy King Street had not shared her wisdom. We talk, on days I'm headed to school, and I discover she's from Philadelphia. "That's where Dad worked!" "Where 'bouts?" "Eerie Avenue, Allegheny Avenue." "I *lived* on Allegheny Avenue!" So we decide we're home girls. Lillian now distributes religious tracts to anybody who'll take them, but once she hears I'm not interested — "Your smile does more good than any piece of paper" — she never pushes.

The Moon in the Water

In my opinion, Lillian is Kuan Yin incarnate. After all, doesn't Kuan Yin sit all day too, one knee drawn up? Okay, Lillian's knee is too stiff to draw up and her ankles too puffy, but she knows what's what. Lillian used to work as a caregiver for the old and confused and has learned not to contradict a whacky narration: "And when they says the sky is falling, you just goes and gets the broom and helps 'em prop it up."

Armed for car-key days with my new advice from Kuan Yin—"Get into the fiction!"—I learn more about Kintnersville (where the goat is still living, this afternoon) and Juliustown (where George is awaitin', this very hour). "Over by McElven's garage?" "No, no, up by the ice plant." Car-key days operate as if somebody popped out the tape "Marvin at eighty," which had been running smoothly, and slipped in the tape "Marvin at twenty," crisp as ever. Without sleep, he looks more and more cadaverous as a car-key day wears on, but now that I'm smarter, I don't worry as much that he might try to stand up and hunt for the car keys himself. I can distract him with the map of south Jersey and weave in an alternate story, "George called and said Elbert is going to pick him up."

At their worst, car-key days plagued us about once every three weeks. Finally, instead of worsening, they disappeared altogether for his last few months. His mind did occasionally run another kind of tape, one that I initially mistook for car-key lurches back toward his youth, but which I soon interpreted as a sneak preview. By then he was too weak to contemplate stepping out to hunt for anything, and in a tone not at all nervous and car-keyed-up, he'd say, "Elbert is waitin' on me" or "Kath, are you ready now to walk me over to that staircase?" We have no staircase. "Yeah, pretty soon." "Okay." Or, on another day, he'd say, "I think I'll just sit on this first step awhile." His mind seemed to be sending him not visions out of the past but views of the future, metaphors for the move into spirit: stepping up, climbing onto another floor in a house of many floors. Maybe he's getting a better glimpse than I past the soot on this scroll.

What'd You Say, Kuan?

A tenth-century ink and tinted drawing shows a male
Water-Moon Kuan Yin on a rocky bank by a pond.
Overlooking an abundant supply of lotuses, he sits up
straight with his right leg folded and right foot tucked
under his left knee. He holds a long willow whisk in one
hand, a water jar in the other. His long hair trails down
from behind his ears in two braided ponytails, then the
clasps let some looser strands flow over his shoulders.
From three-quarter view, only one ear shows, and it looks
unusually long; what's the matter with that ear? Strands
of topaz festoon the ear, upper arms, bare chest. A big red
circle—halo? moon?—almost completely encloses him and
his rock. Only his left foot hangs outside this curve, resting
on a yellow lotus bloom. On the top left of the drawing,
three tiny people on a cloud kneel toward Kuan Yin, but
the bubble shuts them out.

After a car-key bout of sleeplessness, Dad has snoozed
for almost two solid days, and when he wakes up, he is
rested, calm, and sensible, but—a big but—he can't hear
a word I'm saying. "You've lost your voice!" Dad exclaims
sympathetically. Although there is obviously something
wrong with his right, "good ear," I let him go on thinking

I have laryngitis, because this interpretation prevents any sighting toward the grimness of total deafness. I call his primary-care physician, and she speculates maybe he's had a small stroke that has affected his hearing? If so, there is nothing to be done.

We resort to notes on a yellow pad: EGGS FOR SUPPER? The rag doll Will lies in a despondent heap, complaining that his little voice cannot pipe loud enough and regretting that he has never learned to write. Not that Dad can read much better. He was a dyslexic learner, I suspect, in days with no such word, and the amount of concentration to decipher thick pen strokes for rocky bank from thin, feathery strokes for willow whisk is just too tiring. I worry not only that he'll miss some specific information but also that he'll curl up as despondently as Will if he's too isolated in his own silent bubble.

So I call his physician again and plead that I think the problem can't be a stroke—no other symptoms—and venture to guess "earwax," of which he has always produced an abundant supply. It's very hard to bring him in to the office now, though, I explain. He's too unsteady to segue from wheelchair to cab; the Handi-Van will hoist the wheelchair, but the van meanders for so long that he'll need to be changed while we're out, and he'll just perfume the van. . . . She gets my point and decides, "I'll come Saturday."

The yellow pad blooms out with the exciting news, DR. COMING TO CLEAN EARS SAT.! On the big day, she's

The Moon in the Water

a little late. She calls to say she hasn't found the syringe yet; the one at the office stays hooked up to something, and this detached one hasn't seen use in a while. But soon she arrives in her weekend togs: slacks, plaid shirt with sleeves rolled up, and two enormously long, salt-and-pepper braids. (Usually her hair is coiled up elegantly on her head.) She carries a huge syringe that looks for all the world like the cake-decorating squirt gun our neighbor back in Cinnaminson used to have, running a catering business out of her basement. Well, we'll see what we can cook up.

Dad sits obligingly on the edge of the bed. We gather basins, warm water, cloths. The doctor squirts some water in the right ear, to a slight flinch; out comes a big collection of brown earwax, like topaz. Dad looks impressed. For good measure, she flushes out the other ear. Is it going to stay the lone stone-deaf one or not?

"Can you *believe* this amazing doctor has just made a *house call*?" I ask in an ordinary tone of voice to test his hearing (though I'd just as soon shout it from the lanai).

"I believe it," he grins.

Weak as Water

Here's another Water-Moon Kuan Yin almost completely enclosed by a halo, with only one foot hanging outside the circle. These artists' schools really did believe in copying their predecessors, with minimal innovation. This sample differs from the preceding one only in that the right leg crosses *over* the left knee instead of under it, and the rocky bank fronts a stream instead of a pond. Don't they get tired of the picture repeating?

When I glance in Dad's room, I see a long, lanky leg hanging way out of the bed. "Better glue me in," Dad says. Next thing I know, the foot has fallen out of its prescribed scope again and—*clunk*—the rest of the body has tumbled after it, onto the carpet. We check his bones and nothing seems to be broken. Although it's Sunday afternoon, I hear hammering in the next apartment and discover two strapping young workers, willing to take time out to lift an old man back into bed.

After this adventure, I rent a hospital bed. Dad has a hard time getting used to its sides. Psychologically, they spell "cage." If he's in a car-key mood, he will try to wriggle over the foot of the bed. Confinement spurs this weak-as-water elder to new feats. *Clunk.* We check his bones and nothing seems to be broken. I put a pillow under his head to go hunt the neighbors. Fortunately, Jed, from the top floor, and his wife, whose name I missed, agree to help: elevator acquaintances pressed into service. They kneel down, calculate leverage, and heave him back into bed.

Next, Dad and I negotiate the policy on bars. I ask, "Do you think it would be safer today to put the sides up?" Sometimes he says, "I think it'd be safer to put them up." If he sees he has say in the decision, he stays put. Sometimes he even delegates, "I think today you had better make the decisions." When I promise to lower the side "if you change your mind," he assesses ruefully, "What mind?" I try to be aware when he's not car-key-antsy and put the sides back down.

Eventually, we haven't had the sides up for one whole year; he's calmer awake and less mobile in his sleep. But one night I hear a *clunk* at 3 a.m. He's fallen onto the carpet. We put a pillow under his head and check his bones, which seem to be unhurt. Who to call?

Nora, the nurse, has explicitly offered, "Call me anytime, day or night." I call her and Ed, the manager. This by-now-familiar rough sketch of elder-lifting yields a new glow. First Nora, and then Ed, promptly respond, "Oh, I'll be right there." Not even a hint of annoyance, not

a moment's hesitation to remind me how unwelcome it is to
be called at 3 a.m.! "Oh, I'll be right there." Once back in
bed, Dad gives them an amazing, bright smile. He knows
his life is dashing on, like a stream, out of my picture,
but weak water can dissolve mountains and find sea—no
problem, says Kuan.

Moon Wears Out

Kuan Yin hangs onto a rock on her island, peering into the water for a reflection of the moon. The moon is a squashed ball, then half a watermelon slice, then a pale fingernail paring. Its reflection in the water gets more and more diaphanous.

Will obligingly starts to wear out apace with Dad, just so he can keep up as an *akamai* conversationalist, *knowledgeable*. "Marv! Old age is for the birds!" Will exclaims. "My arm's wearing out." He holds out a limb where the cotton stuffing shows through. "That's what comes from good livin' and hard huggin'," Will explains. "Yeah?" "But," says Will, "do you think I'm going to give up huggin'? No way!" Will gives Dad a hug: "If all that huggin' wears out my arms, well, then, so be it!"

Next thing that wears out is Will's nightshirt. He's had this blue striped rectangle, with three ragged holes for head and arms, a mere fifty years. "Did you make that?" Dad asks. "Maybe Gram." Gram did sew some doll clothes for me; I distinctly remember a purple cotton gown with two rows of lace tacked on for Polly. But we deduce that Gram could not have made Will's nightshirt because all Gram's creations carried precise hems, and Will's shirt has been frayed from the start. Ergo, made by Kath. "She's going to make me a new one," Will says hopefully.

Finally I relent and concoct Will a new nightshirt, out of a round of cloth that somebody cut with pinking shears and tied with a ribbon on top of a jar of homemade liliko'i jam. Will's new jam-jar nightshirt has three raggedy holes, just like the old one. By sewing the two halves of a snap on the back, I exhaust my domestic skills.

Will chatters on about the new nightshirt. He explains that its white flowers make it an aloha shirt, "just like Marv's"—pointing to the aloha shirt that Marv has on at that very moment, with white flowers and blue background in exactly the same shade. "I knew if I picked out a new nightshirt in this color and pattern, I'd be at the *height of fashion*, just like Marv," Will explains. This line about height of fashion makes Dad laugh. In Will's youth, Dad wore work pants he'd patched himself, with randomly colored thread, and thin cotton shirts speckled with paint jobs past. Ironing them back then, I watched them grow more and more diaphanous.

Next Will's foot wears out, "from all that dancin' I do." I sew up his foot, but his stuffing-gaped arms are impervious to stitches: not enough "skin" left. "Marv! I'm worn to a frazzle," Will complains; "I never knew what a 'frazzle' was, but I think it's *us*!" Next day, Will reports, "Marv! Today another thread fell out of my nose!" Back at Will's origin, Dad had sewn Will a tidy triangle of a nose.

Now his fine schnozzle is down to one thread. "Old age is so *insulting*," Will opines.

Of course, age has its compensations. One auspicious day a single wisp stands up on Will's head. "Marv! My hair is growing back!" "He never had hair," Dad reminds us. "That's irrelevant," Will says. "I'm not going to be bald anymore. You can *see* I'm finally getting hair."

Despite Will's fragile state, he does a yeoman's job helping Marv, as *he* wears out. To change Dad's diaper, I need him to turn first on his left side, then on his right. With a heroic lurch, he turns to the left. But—no more energy for the second turn. ("Rolling" him has never worked, as Dad resists automatically, with surprising strength.) So Will dashes over: "I'll help you, Marv!" I lay Will on his stomach by the rail on the right. "Okay, I'm hangin' on, Marv! I'm savin' you a spot at the rail," Will pipes. Dad turns halfway. Since Will's rudimentary nightshirt still gapes at the back, he obligingly makes himself look as comical as possible. Dad deigns to smile at Will's antics. "Help Will!" I urge.

Dad, as a Kuan Yin always willing to help out, makes a gargantuan effort to turn to Will.

One more turn, today. One more, tomorrow. Then—no more.

一花五葉開
一葉一如来
知誓是深海
回回運苦財
仁治壬寅歳
九月初一日
門　道元賛

Moon Sealed Red (1)

In a woodblock print called "Kannon on a Lotus Leaf,"
Kuan Yin floats at "royal ease," under the Japanese name
and in a male form. An enormous leaf makes a streamlined
boat. Bundles of leaf fiber sidle up to bundles of waves,
and strands of wavy hair drip over his shoulder: everything
reflecting everything else. Propping himself on an arm, he
folds a leg flat, in well-drawn perspective. He has pulled
up the other leg and drapes a beautiful hand over the knee.
The background paper is brown and blotchy, like a lunch
bag that got caught in the rain.

Remember that narrow ledge where Water-Moon
Kuan Yin peered out at the bay? In print after print, the
overhang looked hacked, eaten out by wave and wind.
The precariousness announced, clearly enough, that this
perch would one day let loose. Dad's "one day" came on 24
February 2006, when he died at home, after almost five
years here.

This particular woodblock print of Kannon dates from
the fifteenth century, but the curator tells us that artists
have copied it several times, from pictures in China.
Apparently, this falling off ledges happens over and over.
When Dad got past the initial shock of the move over the
precipice from New Jersey to Hawai'i, he concluded, "It's

lucky I landed out here with you!"—as if Kuan Yin had picked him up bodily and tossed him over the waves, a beanbag dad. He kept slipping down further notches. After a fall in April 2004, he abandoned his walker. By June 2004, he could no longer sit up at the table and concentrate long enough to put his jigsaw puzzles together. He pronounced mildly, "Well, you just have to let go of some things."

On February 24, Simmy (our amazing helper for the past nineteen months) was here in the morning, and the hospice nurse, Cindy, came by—for the first time—at 4 p.m. When she heard that Dad's urine had stopped the afternoon before and his bowels were emptying out, she exclaimed, "Hon, he's going!" She hopped in her car, despite rush-hour traffic, to get a prescription for morphine, in case Dad panicked at fluid filling his lungs. (He never panicked, though you could hear the congestion rattling all day.) This Kuan Yin from hospice then cajoled her boss on this Friday afternoon to agree to a "courtesy pronouncement" over the weekend: a visit from their nurse to confirm the death and to call the mortuary, bypassing 911 and the hoopla. Cindy also persuaded a Kuan Yin of a pharmacist to dispense the peacock-blue morphine: "Oh, I trust her to pay; I know them!" Still, Cindy only gave Dad the first, experimentally small dose before she left. It was approaching the time for me to give a second dose when he died at 8:05 p.m., totally lucid.

The whole top half of "Kannon on a Lotus Leaf" is covered with inked characters, and superimposed over the calligraphy hangs a huge red seal. The rim looks like Kuan Yin's visible moon, right there over the boat.

At 6:00, though I knew Dad wasn't swallowing anymore, I asked, "Do you want a *little* bit of cottage cheese and banana?" "That—sounds—*good*!" He ate about two mouthfuls, accommodating as always. At 7:30 I asked, "Would you feel more comfortable if I try to change your diaper?" "Yes." (Conscientious ol' bowels, clearing themselves out.) Though he'd been too weak for a couple of months to help much with the changing, this time he miraculously managed to turn, first on one side, then on the other, so I had the satisfying feeling that we were doing a task together: "Man, we're getting good!" I remember as a young child playing on the cement floor of a mechanic's garage, while Dad and old man McElven, his early mentor, worked silently, companionably, at some car repair job. The mutual respect hung palpably in the air then, as it did now. When I took the basin of water out and returned half a minute later, he had stopped breathing. He was lying, at royal ease, on the second side he'd turned to, and his beautiful hands were folded around the rail.

Over the years, some of the details might fade, but the seal remains, the seal among all these reflecting souls, like the brassy afterimage of Kuan Yin's bright moon.

Moon Sealed Red (2)

Kuan Yin, come sit on your lotus-leaf boat again for a minute, so I can tell this story of Dad's ashes, okay?

A long line of friends helps with the ashes. My neighbor Nora drives me to Nu'uanu on Monday, after the weekend Dad died, to make arrangements for the cremation. Acres and acres of stone markers climb the slopes. On Tuesday, though the rain has started to pelt down, a colleague, Sina, takes me to fetch the ashes, making me feel less guilty about pulling her out in a deluge by exclaiming now and then, "I love rain!" The downpour holds off for a moment just as we arrive, the white mists swathing the mountains. I've brought a muslin bag, printed in international words for peace, so I can put the box of ashes inside and have my hands free for the rail. As I pause to gaze at markers from the early 1900s and heft the bag to my shoulder, it occurs to me that Dad would have been carrying me, many years before, when I had exactly the same earthly weight that he now has. The circularity mesmerizes me.

I plan to scatter the ashes in the ocean, but I'm

stymied by an unusual spell of heavy rains: forty days and forty nights, as the weathercasters all dredge up the biblical phrase. Next a sewer main breaks, spilling millions of gallons of raw sewage off Waikīkī beach. Recriminations for ignoring warning signs fly.

Finally, on May 25, three months after Dad died, a colleague Judith, the elements, the dispersed mess, and I are all ready to release his ashes. Judith pulls up at 7 a.m. in a tiny sports car, top down, a yellow surfboard with its nose poking between the front seats and its tail flaunting out the back. Wedged next to its curve, I have the momentary feel of riding a dolphin. I can almost hear Will mutter, back in the apartment, "How come Marv gets to go surfing and I'm stuck at home?"

We drive past touristy Waikīkī to a small beach at Kahala. The beach is almost empty, a few homeless folks sitting in the shelter. The sky is incredibly blue, and the water is incredibly clear. I expect to see waves creaming up on the sand, but this water is flowing parallel to the beach at a good clip, blue ripples cupping gold light. Very far out, two tiny fishermen stand perfectly still on reefs, at the left and right edges of our field of vision: Kuan Yin's two companions over the waves.

As we undo the ties on the bag of ashes and the bag of rose petals (loose, so there's no string from a lei to interfere with fish), a passerby, out for a walk, comes into view. It turns out she's retired from the university. Judith half-recognizes her from committee work: "I admired your orientation class for freshmen." The woman says she now teaches an exit workshop for students called "Passages." She has obviously arrived appropriately, so we invite her to join us.

The Passerby agrees and stands with Judith while I read a few lines praising Marvin: "He was a dignified, patient, and considerate old guy. As Will would say, 'Marv, you're going to be a hard act to follow!' Now it's time to relinquish the physical remnants of this earthly incarnation back to the natural elements. His spirit is already free." I conclude with the two lines I've used as meditation the past few months, "As the beautiful soul of Marvin delights the spirits, may peace and peace and peace be everywhere." Because this meditation goes all the way back to Dad's death, I choke up on the last line.

Judith gives me a hug, then wades into the water in this shallow area, pushing the surfboard as it floats the heavy, plastic bag of ashes. That form for Kuan Yin looks as calm headed out on a yellow board as the form looked on a lotus leaf. When the water reaches Judith's waist, she scatters the petals first. Even at this distance, their brilliant red glows on the blue water. Then Judith casts slow handfuls of ashes. Stretching themselves out in the air, they catch the morning light, float down to join the petals. Each gauze of ash looks amazingly free, exuberant.

The Passerby cries too. Her memories are hers, mine are mine, but we're all Passersby.

Oh, and Kuan Yin? Before you take those red petals out of sight, fill in how we got to the point of choosing the ashes.

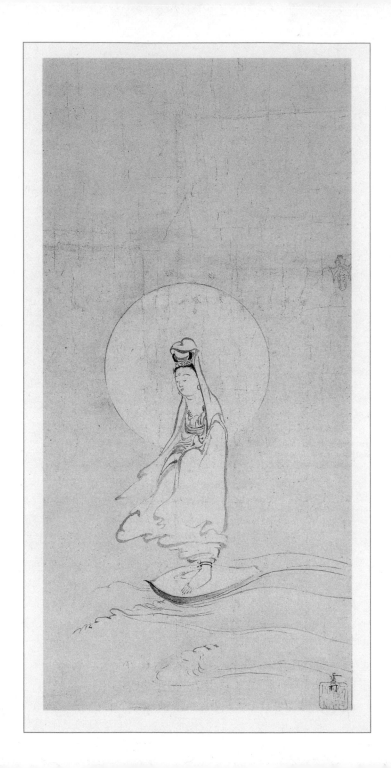

Kuan Yin Not Contained in a Box

According to an old story, Water-Moon Kuan Yin
floated into Chiang-yin harbor on a big lotus petal. With
concentrated moonbeams playing all around her, she
paddled up to a boat. The boatman, however, frightened at
the apparition, tried to push it away with an oar. A painting
now memorializes this event, sketching Kuan Yin with
tightly clutched jar and moon-haloed head. The painting
doesn't show the oarsman, but tiny calligraphy records
his folly. The writing tattles that he shoved the lotus petal
away three times, until finally Kuan Yin, holding her small
jar high out of reach of the flailing oar, shouted across the
waves, "Cut it out! Do you want this gift or not?"

Dad's presents over the years never followed the
automatic trigger of Christmas or birthday. A package
would arrive in Hawai'i whenever the spirit moved him.
He'd bake a loaf of bread and mail it, dry by its arrival—
though still good toasted. Sometimes he'd put packages of
lemon tea in the box or a couple of apples. But surely the
strangest gift he sent was a snapshot of a large, homemade,
wooden box on a sawhorse, labeled with the words, "Here is
the coffin you asked for."

Did I ask for a coffin? Whose coffin? Could father-daughter relations have soured without my noticing? My health seemed excellent. I had aged only into my thirties. Yet he had evidently built me an old-time coffin, the top widening out to cuddle shoulders, then tucking in around the head. Was this abandoned dad in New Jersey wishing me to the devil? Here was a gift I might push away with my oar.

As I suspiciously inspected the photo, it came back to me that I had officiated at this coffin's launch after all. At about seventeen, hearing for the first time of the high cost of burials—all brass, plush, and pomp—I fulminated to Dad about this rip-off industry: thousands of dollars for a hole in the ground. I wound up my peroration by proposing, "Why, you could make me a coffin out of scrap boards for *nothing*!" It didn't occur to me that it might cost *something* for him to picture burying his teenage child, as Grandpa H. had personally dug the hole for his three-year-old during the 1918 influenza epidemic, when the undertakers—and his wife—were all too sick to notice whose baby died. Dad didn't comment on my critique of the mortuary business, no doubt taking all such images of burials, swank or humble, and pushing them away with an oar.

Yet almost two decades later, here comes this image of my coffin, along with, yes, a gift: the realization that he had listened to his teen, taken her seriously, and remembered her proposal. Aware that he wouldn't always be around to carry out the request (Mom had died by then), he finally

The Moon in the Water

sawed and nailed the boards together, for my future, simple, un-ripped-off burial, weird apparition though it was.

When Dad moved to Hawai'i, he asked whether I would be shipping his body back to the family cemetery plot in New Jersey, or whether I would be cremating him here, "like that good friend of yours." That good friend, Joe, died in 1992. Joe's partner, Clifford, hired a boat and took some friends out in the dusk to scatter his ashes. He asked if we would each dip ash—from a cardboard box—into the ocean, along with white gardenias, leaping out of themselves with redolence and longing. "Ashes to ashes" had previously conjured for me something gray and powdery, paper ash really, but these ashes were beige and heavy, like beach sand, with white flecks of bone, like shell. It stunned me—the great generosity that Clifford would offer us the gift of somehow touching that body, each levering ash.

"Well," I answered Dad, "I'd just as soon scatter your ashes here, but I'll ship your body if you want to use that cemetery lot Grandpa gave us." By the time Grandpa bought the lots, he must have been long reconciled to Dad as son-in-law, though he had refused to attend the wedding. Basing his judgment solely on Dad's grammar (which my computer program now similarly dismisses in hysterical squiggles of red and gray), the old man had warned my mom, "Your children will be idiots!" That grandfather died a few months before I graduated valedictorian, a small-town affair, which I would nevertheless have liked to see vindicating my dad (and all squiggled grammar) to fuddy-duddies. Now that I mention to Dad his place among grandfather's carefully ordered cemetery lots, Dad grunts, "I ain't liable to miss it. You can scatter my ashes here."

I did test out my coffin once, on a trip back to New Jersey. It fit. Much later, when Dad moved here and we emptied his house, I spotted the heavy, disassembled boards under the eaves in the attic, looking like helpful planks over the beams. I left the planks there. Like Dad and Kuan Yin, I'll take the fire and the water—not that I have anything against the good, crumbling earth.

Afterword

In the Buddhist tradition, Water-Moon Kuan Yin has many meanings, with different moods felt by different viewers:

1. Like the reflection of the moon in the water, our plans, successes, worries, romances, and identities fool us into thinking they have grand importance. Some commentators look at this fleetingness and decide they ought to disdain life. Play it safe; don't get attached!

2. Other Buddhists, however, far from disdaining the reflection of the moon in the water, try to appreciate those fleeting plans and people: the glittery shapes of each valuable moment. Still, they try not to mistake the shimmers in the pond for the ultimate reality or happiness-maker, the moon. Rejoice as the shapes come out on a bright night; rejoice as they go, on a dark, velvety night.

3. As the moon can show up in many bodies of water, even a puddle, so too does a bodhisattva lodge hidden in everyone. Buddhist philosopher Yung-chia Hsüan-chüeh taught in the seventh century, "One moon reveals universally all water, and all water universally contains one moon" (quoted in Chün-fang Yü, *Kuan-yin: The Chinese Transformation of Avalokiteśvara* [New York: Columbia University Press, 2001] 237). Light can manifest to all through all. Recognize every experience as potentially a teacher.

4. Does the moon circle Kuan Yin or does she project a halo from herself? Inner light and outer light are the same. They're both ripples in the water from an unstoppable source. Everything is interdependent. Be moon, or be Kuan Yin, to each other.

5. As the moon floats at hand in the water, so too is enlightenment available. Ch'an (Zen) commentators add, there is no need for a long struggle or bookish apprenticeship to rise to the skies. Just wake up and reflect the moon now.

Sources for Art Works
Described or Reproduced

Some of the paintings I mention are general descriptions, but others are very specific, found in the following sources. When I drew from a picture, I took only a few of the artist's hints and mixed in Dad's life. Quotations are also cited here.

Dug Up Kuan Yin, page 1
"Water-Moon Kuan Yin" on a stele, dated 1096 C.E., found in an excellent book by Chün-fang Yü, *Kuan-yin: The Chinese Transformation of Avalokiteśvara* (New York: Columbia University Press, 2001), 243–44. I am also grateful to Professor Yü for telling me which of her pictures are inaccessible in temples and which are catalogued in museums, so I might query about them.

Pilgrim Gifts, page 4
This picture is by Chao I, dated 1313. Courtesy of the National Palace Museum, Taipei, Taiwan, Republic of China.

Water Pill, page 8
Water and Moon Kuan-yin (Shui-yueh Kuan-yin), Chinese, late thirteenth–early fourteenth century. Hanging scroll, ink, slight color and gold on silk, 43 ¾ x 30 inches (111.12 x 76.20 cm). Courtesy of the Nelson-Atkins Museum of

Art, Kansas City, Missouri. Purchase: Nelson Trust, 49–60. Photograph by Jamison Miller.

The Moon in the Computer, page 11

The epigraph is from the *Great Prajñā-pāramitā Sūtra,* quoted in Yü, *Kuan-yin,* 236.

Waterfall ID, page 14

I saw this picture in a journal called *Sekai bijutsu zenshu* (Tokyo, 1965): 99.

Yankee Moon, page 21

I describe a picture from Yü, *Kuan-yin,* 96: the frontispiece of the *Fo-shuo Kuan-shih-yin chiu-k'u ching,* printed and donated by Imperial Concubine Cheng between 1573 and 1615. The upside-down bird in this drawing must be a version of the kind of diving bird that appears in the illustration for "Pilgrim Gifts."

For a picture of my dad with his Yankee screwdriver, see also "Moon Rings," 90.

Transferring the Willow, page 25

Ink and color on silk, dated 943 c.e., found in Cornelius P. Chang, "Kuan-Yin Paintings from Tun-Huang: Water-Moon Kuan-Yin," *Journal of Oriental Studies* 15.2 (1977), 147–48 and Plate 1. The painting has a male Kuan Yin, with a mustache, but I changed the Kuan Yin in my story to female.

Willy Moon, page 29

Frontispiece of the *Pai-i Ta-pei wu-yin-hsin t'o-lo-ni ching,* dated 1603, in Yü, *Kuan-yin,* 95, 97.

Artsy Crappy Moon, page 32

I saw the picture I describe, "Kannon with Willow Branch," at an exhibit at the Honolulu Academy of Arts in 2002.

That hanging scroll, with colors on silk, came from Hōjuin Temple, Japan, and is originally from Korea, Koryō period (918–1392 c.e.).

Since the scroll was so hard to see through the soot, I made up my own picture. Will is in the middle, and Dad is in the wheelchair. I took the liberty of giving Kuan Yin's usual high headpiece a hat brim and a feather lei, and I gave her a shower-tree sprig instead of a willow branch.

Moon Body, page 37

I saw this Kuan Yin picture once in the Asian Art Museum, Seattle, and am writing from memory and from my scribbled notes of the visit.

Kuan Yin Prescription, page 39

The quotations in the first paragraph are from Yü, *Kuan-yin*, 237–38.

Riding the Tides in the Handi-Van, page 44

I saw this tenth-century poster, called "Kuan Yin Appears in Twenty-Four Manifestations," in Yü, *Kuan-yin*, 230. She says it's originally from *Zuzōbu*, volume 6 of the Taishō Tripitaka.

For my picture, I put the two Water-Moon Kuan Yins from the top corners of the poster side by side, on their cupcake-shaped rocks. I turned the Kuan Yins into passengers, waiting for the Handi-Van to come back. The Xerox of my dad's official Handi-Van card shows up the little moon ring over his face very well. The two Chinese characters at the bottom say "water" and "moon."

Peace Moon, page 50

My drawing is more or less based on the same tenth-century poster, called "Kuan Yin Appears in Twenty-Four

Manifestations," in Yü, *Kuan-yin*, 230. This time I drew a
portion of the eleven-headed Kuan Yin from the center of
the poster. I tried to put the heckler on the bicycle in one of
her hands. The elephant trumpeting is also from the poster;
here it's the approving car horns.

Moon Passing through Cloud, page 54
> "Moon in Water," twelfth century, in Yü, *Kuan-yin*, 246.
> For a picture of my dad tossing flowers from a box at Elbert's
> memorial service, see the drawing for "Artsy Crappy Moon,"
> 32.

Blue Moon, page 56
> The inspiration was the same picture I used in the preceding
> vignette, from Yü, *Kuan-yin*, 246.

Calling the Moon, page 60
> The account in the first paragraph of a lost Kuan Yin
> painting is from Chang, "Kuan-Yin Paintings," 146.

Accidental Moons, page 68
> The account of these three paintings is found in Robert La
> Thorp and Richard Ellis Vinograd, *Chinese Art and Culture*
> (Upper Saddle River, NJ: Prentice Hall, and New York:
> Harry Abrams, 2001), 276–77. This scrimshaw sits on
> my desk. I suddenly noticed that the artist, Paul Sheldon
> of Honolulu, must have been inspired by the same three
> paintings that inspired "Accidental Moons." By putting the
> crane in Kuan Yin's lap and letting the monkey peer over her
> shoulder, Paul has made the composition distinctively his
> own. The photograph is by Joseph Singer.

Roundabout Moon, page 78
> "White-Robed Kannon," by Kanō Kōi, c. 1569–1636,
> hanging scroll, ink on paper, in Stephen Little, *Visions of
> the Dharma: Japanese Buddhist Paintings and Prints in the*

Honolulu Academy of Arts (Honolulu: Honolulu Academy of Arts, 1991), 158–59.

Kuan Yin's Taxable Domain, page 81

I again describe a picture from Yü, *Kuan-yin,* 96: the frontispiece of the *Fo-shuo Kuan-shih-yin chiu-k'u ching,* printed and donated by Imperial Concubine Cheng between 1573 and 1615.

Slim Pickings/Fat Moon, page 86

The directions to artists for painting Kuan Yin's halo and nimbus are found in Chang, "Kuan-Yin Paintings," 151. The pointy, broken bamboo are pictured in his Plate 1.

Moon Rings, page 90

I describe "Nyoirin Kannon," or "Jewel-Holding, Wheel-Turning Avalokiteshvara (Kannon)," early Muromachi period, fifteenth century, ink, colors, and gold on silk, printed in Little, *Visions of the Dharma,* 60–61.

Inspired by this hanging scroll, I drew my dad with six hands, holding his tools and Jonette's bicycle wheel, and wearing his railroad cap.

Kuan Yin Foot Dangler, page 95

The information on chloroplasts and mitochondria is from Lewis Thomas, *The Lives of a Cell* (New York: Bantam, 1974), 2, 82.

ER Moon, page 98

"White-robed Kannon Seated on a Rock," Kamakura period, early thirteenth century, ink on paper.

This hanging scroll belongs to the Alsdorf collection of Japanese painting and is printed here by kind permission of Marilynn Alsdorf. I am also grateful to Barbara Pope and Maureen Liu-Brower of Barbara Pope Book Design for generously preparing the scan.

Car-Key Kuan, page 107

This is the same scroll I describe for "Artsy Crappy Moon," pages 32–33.

What'd You Say, Kuan?, page 111

This Water-Moon Kuan Yin is from the Tun-Huang caves, described in Chang, "Kuan-Yin Paintings," 148 and Plate 3.

Moon Sealed Red (1), page 120

"Kannon on Lotus Leaf," woodblock print, Muromachi period, c. fifteenth century, Honolulu Academy of Arts, Gift of James A. Michener, 1991 (24,600). Used by permission.

Kuan Yin Not Contained in a Box, page 128

The story of the apparition is modified from Yü, *Kuan-yin*, 255–56. The picture is "One-petal Kannon," or "The Bodhisattva Kannon Crossing the Sea on a Lotus Petal," ink on paper, Muromachi period, by Zen artist Sesson Shūkei (1504–1589?). This hanging scroll belongs to the Alsdorf collection of Japanese painting and is printed here by permission of Marilynn Alsdorf. I am also grateful to Barbara Pope and Maureen Liu-Brower of Barbara Pope Book Design for preparing the scan.